D1040888

Inside Poop

America's leading colon therapist
defies conventional medical wisdom
about your health and well-being

by Scott W. Webb

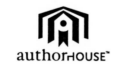

authorHOUSE™

1663 LIBERTY DRIVE, SUITE 200
BLOOMINGTON, INDIANA 47403
(800) 839-8640
WWW.AUTHORHOUSE.COM

© 2006 Scott W. Webb. All Rights Reserved.

No part of this book may be reproduced, stored in a retrieval system, or transmitted by any means without the written permission of the author.

First published by AuthorHouse 12/29/05

ISBN: 1-4259-0211-1 (sc)

Library of Congress Control Number: 2005910232

Printed in the United States of America
Bloomington, Indiana

This book is printed on acid-free paper.

Disclaimer

I have performed hundreds of colonics on myself and experienced tremendous benefits. I have assisted others with internal cleansing including my two teenagers, my mother, my sister, my friends, and hundreds of clients without injury. I would hope that you have a similar experience with internal hygiene.

This book describes personal experiences which might not be safe for you to do yourself at home. Therefore, consult your doctor before taking any action which might affect your health.

This information is for educational purposes only. It is not intended as advice for self diagnosis or a prescription for self treatment. Any adverse effect arising directly or indirectly from this material is not the responsibility of the author, publisher, distributors, or bookstores.

The intent of this book is to stimulate thought and to encourage optimism regarding the benefits of a healthy lifestyle.

Scott W. Webb

*This book is dedicated
to the hip kids of the
younger generation including
Arthur and Madeleine.*

Special Thanks!

Thanks first to my brother, Guy Avery, who introduced me to systems thinking and genuine spirituality. I once was so, so, blind.

My parents, Herb and Barbara, also taught me about that systems stuff and "following dreams" in their own amazing ways. And we survived the rubber hitting the road. I would include in that -- Tucker, Cheri, and Rob, and Beth, Terri, and Steve.

Thanks to my ex-wife, Laurie. You are awesome in countless ways including flowing in the language of music. I could not have asked for a better partner in adventure. I do appreciate you returning my vacuum cleaner last week.

Maryglenn, you awaken the giant within. Kentucky should be proud to call you its own. Maryalice, you do likewise. Janie and Alicia, you're cool too.

To my landlord, Mr. Jones -- I see you coming and going and know you are a kind-hearted hero. Thanks for giving me a chance to be your tenant. Another unsung hero of Nashville is Patricia Martin. Thanks to Lee and to Chelsea, both great teachers. And I will always appreciate the wisdom of Bill Page, the teacher's teacher.

Kudos to other pioneers, like Kevin Trudeau, who have braved the way ahead. Same goes to stores like the old Sunshine Grocery, the new Wild Oats, and Whole Foods and to America's good stewards of healthy eating -- Ma, Pa, and Nell Newman.

Thanks to all the folks who suffered through my youth before I knew what I wanted to be. If I could contact you all now and apologize for my ignorance, I would. That includes those who put up with me in the great state of Alaska through the 1980s.

K. Cobb, bro, where did you disappear to? Lori P., you too.

Thanks to Brad DeMeulenaere who helped me edit at the last minute. Thanks to Marti for some really fun times and for introducing me to Watertown and Pumpkin Hollow. The folks at Gray Bear and the guys from I.P.S.B. are pretty groovy also.

I appreciate the support from Will and Susan Fischer and from Betsy S. -- your daughter Evelyn is a high-skipper if ever I have seen one. Last minute thanks to Deborah from McKenzie. Beverly, so glad we're friends. Jewel, Candy, Ken, Jeff, Pam, you too. Brandon -- quit smoking!

Special thanks to my children, Art and Maddie, for sharing cheap living quarters and for helping me to envision a better future for us all. Art created *Inside Poop's* graphic on the cover.

If the readers of this book benefit much, then join with me in appreciating my many fine clients. *Inside Poop* could not have been written without their full cooperation. The faith they entrusted to me and in their own intuition is beyond measure.

Finally, thanks to all the Beat poets who taught me how to write. Craig Bartlett, that includes you. Many of them have passed on now to sit with Indians and other untamed gypsies sharing a peace pipe in the Great Beyond. Jack, save me a place, man.

"The future is here. It's just not widely distributed yet."

William Gibson

Contents

Chapter One
Do you really want to be normal?

When I first became a colon hygienist, I was shocked by the tremendous volume of rotten fecal matter coming out from a typical person. The average release during a cleansing session is three to five feet long. On the extreme end I've seen solid pieces totaling ten feet removed and once witnessed 15 feet of fecal-mess flood from a skinny woman weighing ninety pounds.

One client released 40 feet of fecal matter over the course of five weekly sessions during a two-month juice fast. When she first came it had been three weeks since she had eaten food and eight feet of clay-like poop came out. It left us speechless each successive colonic as we saw eight feet of poop exit weekly (while eating no solid food).

I asked myself, "*Is this normal?* Does this huge volume of inner poop explain why Americans have generally become so ill and dependent on drugs?" I mean drugs for chronic pain, drugs to fall asleep, for depression, sex enhancing drugs, anti-bloating drugs -- you name it. Since I am naturally curious, I began investigating what might cause fecal matter to be held in the gut. Then everywhere I looked, I found answers.

"Does this huge volume of inner poop explain why Americans have generally become so ill and dependent on drugs?"

The starting point, for me, was to ask: "What happens when people start eliminating this excessive fecal matter?" My observation has been that they got better -- feel better, look better, see positive results. Most curious to me has been the total ignorance and denial of this reality by the American medical system.

So we are looking at a health topic filled with curiosities.

My goal in writing this book is to make something perfectly

clear -- America is in danger from an evil *within*. This inner sludge is torturing and killing people now. All the military forces in the world cannot protect us from it. Whoever was supposed to protect us has gone to sleep. Our best watchdog has become retarded, chasing its own tail.

No matter what the health experts instruct us to do, the truth is that the human body can't be sustained by the typical American diet. If you are poor, you eat mostly reconstituted grease and sugar; and if affluent, you eat mostly reconstituted grease and sugar with a sprig of parsley on the side.

Try to eat healthy and you can't. Most salmon ordered in a restaurant today provides no health benefits. Each bite sliced from a slab of gray protein dyed pink is from an animal fed on a diet of antibiotic-laden pellets swimming in a cramped sea water pen. You are too good for that, my friend. Let the other guy or gal eat it while you escape out the back door.

To be wealthy and lose your health seems almost an impossibility, but it's so common that it's become status quo in America. Prosperity should mean <u>function</u> and <u>pleasure</u> without reaching for a pill bottle. So let the other guy eat all that bacon, fries, food-to-go on a bun, and cellophane-wrapped cakes. Chicken raised in a crowded concentration camp isn't fit for consumption either. Deep down you know it's true.

A friend said the other day, "Isn't it awesome that you can get a walnut and apple salad from the drive-thru?" "Yeah," I replied, "If you enjoy eating anti-browning chemicals, preservative waxes, and artificial flavors." You know the fast food industry prides itself on uniformity while apples are anything but uniform in taste. My guess is that apple salad comes laced with a powdered "apple-fresh" flavoring that's murder on the human liver.

You've watched those scary movies where a girl cracks open a door with an ugly monster behind it. You think: "Oh no!" Well, that's how I feel about people's health, knowing as I do what rots inside of them. So -- I will state my findings about this as simply and clearly as possible without jargon or pretensions. In fact, I've considered writing this as a children's book because children are often more open than adults.

And children are the real victims when it comes to the state of things we adults are handing down.

Some people have voiced their opinion that putting water in the colon is not natural, but then do not question if what enters their mouth is natural. *Cheese Nips* don't grow on trees. If you haven't considered that you eat mostly processed food, try eating only uncooked, organic food and notice if your day changes. Eating unconsciously helps to form the unconscious sludge inside.

But no blame here. We've all done it -- I'm just saying, "Get it out!" Using water to flush the colon is actually a hygienic practice as old as civilization. It was addressed in the Dead Sea Scrolls and documented in ancient Egyptian hieroglyphics.

For some people, a mass of poop extends up the entire digestive tract into their liver and the primary side-effect is depression. Other side-effects will be addressed later and it's become big business to those in the medical industry -- a myriad of drugs prescribed and lots of surgeries to remove poisoned, poorly functioning organs.

This subject is potentially gross, but ignoring it does not make it go away. You should know that your predecessors living before the year 1930 did not have this sludge inside of them. Today, the further you go geographically from the U.S., the less this condition exists. America has the distinction of being the planet's toxic bull's-eye. You can track it statistically by the incidence of diverticular diseases of the colon.

Right now your body is doing everything it can to shield itself from this special brand of Twenty-first Century poop-sludge because your insides don't want to touch it any more than you do. It ages you in ways you don't want to age. Dark circles and puffy eyes are a sure sign of it. A flotilla of doctors in white coats telling me (and you) that America does not have a toxicity crisis only makes me bust out laughing.

Groucho Marx already tried that gag years ago when he said, "Who are you going to believe? *Me* or your own eyes?"

As a colonic therapist, I've seen the light.

The time has come to trust your own intuition or suffer the consequences of others making choices for you. Their decisions will fall somewhere on the scale between tragic and moronic. Be aware -- if you mindlessly stick within the system, the statistics are not in your favor. It's difficult for many Americans to grasp that they live within some kind of system.

If it's true that this inside poop does exist, then all the rules about health have changed. That's why you should read this book. The rules have changed.

The cultural condition

A new client sits across from me explaining why she wants to try colonics. She is experiencing chronic yeast infections, daily bloating, and for the past two months she can barely get out of bed from the weight of her feelings of hopelessness, feeling like she has been poisoned.

Heidi has been seen by several doctors over the years and she has only gotten worse. Yet she is attractive, thin, tan, and barely into her 30s. Heidi was raised in Nebraska and this is the impression she projects -- milk and honey, fresh air and sunshine. She has a college degree in finance and there's no doubt she is smart.

"What do you think is wrong with me?" she asks almost pleading for an answer.

I stare back for a second thinking that if I don't write a book about my experiences with colon hygiene, millions of women (and men) just like her will lose their battle to be well. Before I can respond she interrupts: "I've resisted resorting to antidepressants, but I can't go living on like this," she says.

"I know," I reply as we sit again in silence, briefly mourning the loss of her health and the sapping of her basic vitality. The sadness feels overwhelming as I clear my throat. "Well," I begin as she sits upright on the edge of her chair to hear my every word.

"First of all, colon hygiene does not treat illness. By law I can't even address your symptoms." Heidi nods as if to say, "Get on with it."

"You are not the first person I've encountered who has these problems. That means that there is something going on affecting us in general as a culture. So don't take it personally that you are struggling," I explain.

"The fact that you have figured out that colonics might be a solution for you means that you are exceptional," I continue. "The concept of colonics is bizarre. It's not a procedure you can appreciate with your brain, that it could have exceptional benefits, which tells me you're stretching because you truly want to be well."

She smiles.

"Frankly," I add, "Having been through the medical system, you're lucky to have all your body parts left intact."

"Exactly," Heidi nods, "They wanted to give me a hysterectomy."

"Why?" I ask. My mind jumps to another recent client of mine about Heidi's age who did get a total hysterectomy and her gut's symptoms did not improve. When she later complained that she received unnecessary surgery, the doctor told her that "at least she wouldn't need to fear ovarian cancer." And the punch line: because she has no ovaries.

"When young women from our heartland grow cysts on their innards, there's something generally wrong-headed going on."

"I've had cysts on my ovaries," Heidi replies. "I want children so I flat-out told them no-way to surgery. I'm keeping my female parts."

Again I feel incredibly sad. Not for her exactly, but for the entire mess America is in. When young women from our heartland grow cysts on their innards, there's something generally wrong-headed going on.

It was by pure accident that I stumbled into colon hygiene and discovered that it helped people like Heidi get well. So I look at her and say, "There is hope."

Concern is a two-way street

One of the tensions between the medical community and alternative health practitioners is the concern that ordinary people without formal training will start to "practice medicine without a license."

As an alternative health practitioner, I have one response: "I don't want to practice medicine." I want those in medicine to do their job and start helping all these people who come to me and say, "Doctors aren't helping me."

See yourself in history

In 1984 I got married and we had two children fairly quickly. I homeschooled my son for his eighth, ninth, and tenth grades and my daughter for part of the seventh grade. My primary goal was to give them a sense of their place in history.

I met with my daughter, Maddie, as her new homeschool teacher. I wanted to survey her understanding at age twelve. I asked her: "Was the invention of the automobile fifty years ago, one hundred years ago, or five hundred years ago?"

Her reply: "Five hundred years ago?"

I realized that she and I had much ground to cover.

"There exist cultures on the planet today that have low incidence of cancer and heart attacks."

If a person does not understand basic history, he or she will be unable to figure out for themselves what it means to be healthy. One hundred years ago, there were no cell phones, no personal computers, no microwave ovens, no Super Wal-Marts, no drive through restaurants, partly because most people had never driven a car. In 1900 there were also no heart attacks -- none. I believe that the first recorded heart attack was in 1912. Cancer was a minimal threat. As the cause of death then, it was one-in-thirty.

Do you know that there exist cultures on the planet today that have low incidence of cancer and heart attacks? These cultures resemble America one hundred years ago. When people from these cultures move to America, they then get our diseases.

I heard a radiologist speak on her experience treating breast cancer over the past twenty years. When she began her career, she treated mostly women in their fifties, sixties and seventies.

Within two decades that has changed. Her youngest patient now is seventeen. And most of her cancer patients today are in their thirties and forties.

It is important to understand that in the year 1900, American women were not getting breast cancer. They didn't have it in 1776 nor going back to Bible times. It simply is not possible that breast cancer is primarily hereditary in nature. If it were hereditary, that would mean that our ancestors had breast cancer. But they didn't.

It means that something *else* is giving women breast cancer and other cancers in record numbers. If you are a woman in her thirties, it means you better figure out what's going on -- fast. And if you are a man, know that prostate cancer is affecting men younger and younger.

Just before the devastating tsunami hit in Southeast Asia, one man recognized the warning signs and began to run for high ground, encouraging others to join him. Some laughed at what they considered to be paranoia -- and they are no longer with us.

Cancer takes people in a similar fashion. It is abrupt and it is cruel. But cancer is not indiscriminate in who it takes. It can be side-stepped. That is why you don't have the luxury to ignore what is happening around you.

See yourself in history. Recognize the danger signs of the times or you will find yourself a victim of them.

Why you must read this book

A friend told me that my body might have excess yeast growing inside my gut. I discovered two comprehensive books had been written on the subject. I bought both and read them cover to cover.

The books included testimonials, case studies, clinical studies, and proof that Candida yeast had become the cause of many modern disease symptoms. Yet the question remained, "What would I do if I had a yeast problem?"

I would take a pill.

Let's say you have a health problem. Why would you read two books about the subject if the solution is to take a pill? Why not just take the pill?

If you have excess fecal matter in your gut, why read what a colon hygienist has to say on the subject if you can just take a pill? Because there is no such pill.

"Working from the inside-out takes years I regret to say."

I believe in simplicity and taking shortcuts. But this solution requires rolling up your sleeves. Elbow grease gets this job done. Improvement comes immediately, but working from the inside-out takes years I regret to say. And yet, the last thing we think to do is the first thing we should have done. I'll explain that later. Just keep reading.

Know this -- there's no pill coming.

America as one of many civilizations

Back when I was a kid in school, I marveled at the many civilizations which came and went: the ancient Egyptians, the Mayans, the Aztecs. Look at the great stone architecture left behind in Rome and in Greece, the aquifers and coliseums. One of my teachers taught that Rome fell because the people went mad from lead in their water.

I believe that this type of teaching is what kept me on the lookout for some obscure poison which might bring down America. While the media focused on Communist Russia as our enemy, I kept an eye on our water, how it might drive us to insanity. Anyway, I was in the right ball park.

When I became an evangelical Christian as a teen, my focus became on the future. Back in the 1970s, I read all the books on prophesy going around, written by Hal Lindsey and Salem Kirban. I scratched for evidence that America would be there in the end times predicted in the Bible and it wasn't there.

Listening to National Public Radio the other day, I heard that America spends twice the amount on health care of any other nation. The angle on the story was that the reason for this is because prices of services do not fall in line with costs. If a certain procedure or test is more profitable than another, doctors are performing services that are the most profitable.

When I first moved to Tennessee, I had an aversion to the South. Being from Chicago, and living nine years in Alaska, I did not understand Southerners. Therefore, I couldn't find a job to support my wife and two children. I ended up delivering pizza for almost three years. I wore one of those blue caps and drove like a maniac.

One day a customer complained to the manager about their pizza. I did not know the details of the complaint, except that the manager made a big show to the drivers as to how he dealt with complaints. He placed his thumb to his right nostril and blew his nose directly onto the new pizza order.

You could summarize my learning as this: 1) pay attention to what they are putting in the water, 2) learn what makes doctors the greatest profits and avoid those services, especially if it is a surgery, and 3) never complain about your dinner when somebody else is making it and you are not there. Even when you don't complain the ingredients from the food factory might need questioning.

What do these three things have to do with colon hygiene? Everything.

NOW OPEN
in HILLCREST
142 University Ave
Between 2ND & 3rd Avenues

619-578-2909

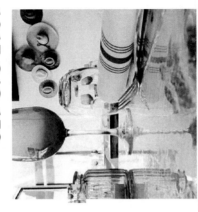

CLANDESTINO
- SEAFOOD & FISH FUSION -

Beach– Styled Seafood with Italian Roots

"**Clandestino** is inspired by Italian coastal cuisine; the menu at this seafood-focused restaurant features everything from lobster bisque and la plancha style octopus entrée, to a crayfish cappellacci fresh pasta dish and LobsBurger (a lobster patty on squid ink bun.)

Several other offerings are also available: Salads, Gluten Free Pastas, Burgers and more.

HOURS
Tue 5:30- 8:30 PM
Wed-Sun 11AM- 8:30PM
HAPPY HOUR
Wed-Sun 4-6 PM

Sunday Brunch
10-2:30 PM

BUY 1 ENTRÉE
(Reg. Price)
Get 2nd Entrée at
50% OFF
Equal or lesser Value
Expires 9/9/16

Catering & Take Out

CHECK OUR
Daily
Seafood Specials!
ASK About
My Palate Choice"

Chapter Two
The beauty of inner health

"A book, written to teach what to do for a cold or a sore throat and which herbs and vitamins to take for a particular malady, doesn't convey the whole truth. I am not interested in remedies for nasal congestion, constipation, heart burn, headaches, allergies, PMS, or pre-menopausal symptoms. For I no longer have any of these problems."

Tonya Zavasta, *Your Right to be Beautiful*

The above quote is one of the most revealing passages written today on health. Allow me to explain:

Tonya Zavasta has overcome her symptoms of disease. All of them. At fifty years old. Her hourglass figure could be envied by college girls. And she says that you can have such vibrancy too -- health and beauty without a remedy for each problem.

I heard Tonya Zavasta speak after an invitation by a friend. I didn't know who she was and I happened to sit in the front row. I bought her book afterwards and shook her hand because she is the real deal. She ties health to beauty and once you get past that, it's obvious that she is right. Illness destroys beauty.

Health, however, radiates it.

Ten years ago I recall thinking, "I am deficient in *some*thing." I went to the health food store and looked at all the supplements. Was it a vitamin, a mineral, an enzyme? Was there an extract that would revitalize me down to my cellular structure?

I never found that perfect miracle supplement and how glad I am now. The whole truth is much better. The whole truth is that health radiates from the inside-out.

I went to the library four years ago and checked out my limit of twenty books, all on the topic of health. I discovered a passage in an obscure book published in 1965 by Adelle Davis called, *Let's Get Well*. At the time I was hunting down the reason my clients were so incredibly backed-up with poop. The discovery also explained why

I had felt lacking down to my cellular level. I had become deficient in bile.

Adelle Davis explains:

"If the amount of bile is insufficient ... fats remain in such large particles that enzymes cannot combine readily with them; hence fat digestion is incomplete and fat absorption markedly reduced.

Part of the undigested fat quickly combines with any calcium and iron in the food to form insoluble soaps; thus these minerals are prevented from reaching the blood, and the hard soaps, causing overly firm stools, bring about constipation. Poor elimination associated with gall-bladder problems invariably indicates a major loss of vital minerals.

Most solid fats obtained in foods quickly melt at body temperature. If little bile is present, this melted, undigested fat coats all foods, preventing enzymes from combining efficiently with proteins and carbohydrates, thus decreasing their digestion.

Intestinal bacteria multiply enormously on this huge mass of undigested food, releasing quantities of histamine and gas, which cause discomfort, halitosis, and a foul-smelling stool. Much undigested food is usually lost in the stools, and becomes a serious problem when the calorie requirements are high and proteins badly needed for repair." (pgs. 179-180)

What does this mean? Quite simply, the quantity of a person's bile alone can determine the quality of their poop. Quality of poop indicates their quality of life. Hard poop plugs up the elimination system which begins a downward health spiral.

There are (at least) three reasons why this could have you saying, "Eureka!"

#1) **Osteoporosis explained**. Americans lead the world in many things, including osteoporosis, or bone loss. In order to prevent it, doctors recommend supplementing calcium, which makes America the world leader in supplementing calcium. And the American Dairy Association recommends eating dairy products, which we do, so we lead the planet in dairy consumption. This appears to be a vicious cycle because all this emphasis on calcium has not improved osteoporosis, which actually has gotten worse in recent years.

The same condition which contributes to osteoporosis, of calcium in food bonding to fats, also creates hard stools in the colon. It's no secret that one of the side effects of calcium supplementation and dairy consumption is constipation.

Adelle Davis has explained why -- *"Undigested fat quickly combines with any calcium and iron in the food to form insoluble soaps; thus these minerals are prevented from reaching the blood, and the hard soaps, causing overly firm stools, bring about constipation."*

Where has all the calcium gone?

If calcium is prevented from reaching the bloodstream under these conditions, there is no way it can reach the bones. If osteoporosis is epidemic in America, then this translates that most Americans are not assimilating calcium into their blood. If Americans are taking, but not assimilating calcium, then *where* is it going?

Calcium combines with iron and fat in food and then forms hard stools. The assumption would be that calcium then exits the body unused, except these "hard soaps" become unpassable. Calcium lines the colon walls in the form of a disgusting bone-like cement which the water of a colonic helps to flush out. Otherwise it just stays there.

#2) **Fiber.** If you are thinking ahead, then you have already reached the conclusion that supplementing fiber to solve constipation misses the cause of hard stools, which is insufficient bile. Taking fiber can be like adding straw to adobe bricks: Calcium/iron + undigested fat + fiber = brick. A major function of the colon is to remove water. In other words, the colon is a kind of poop dehydrator and under the right conditions it can dry and manufacture calcified concrete -- in astounding amounts.

So if your doctor recommends fiber for constipation, like he or she recommends calcium for osteoporosis, then you know he or she has not read "Let's Get Well," published in 1965 and available in your public library. Ask your doctor about this!

#3) **Bile**. Bile is the key. If your liver is not adequately producing bile and you address only the symptoms of illness, you will never get well nor look well.

Connect the dots between food, the liver's production of bile, and constipation. You absolutely cannot be healthy if your colon has become congested with hard soaps. One obvious reason is that this condition results from a daily cycle requiring a healthy, bile-producing liver. If you already realized this, then skip ahead to the next chapter.

Otherwise, understand that every time you eat fat, your food requires bile to digest it. Without sufficient bile, minerals present in your food are combining with fat to form poop that is rock hard. When this poor combination of ingredients passes through twenty feet of small intestine and finally reaches the colon, water gets extracted there. A hamburger at this juncture, for example, would resemble a clenched fist.

Now -- pass that.

Fifty years ago bobby socks and car hops were "in" and the insufficient bile problem was uncommon. Hamburgers were no problem then to digest. Today, most Americans have a serious bile limitation. If you need further proof that low bile production and inner congestion could afflict an entire nation, observe that diseases of the colon would be increasing under these conditions. Did I mention that America leads the world in diverticular disease of the colon and colon cancer? Yes, sadly, by far.

Ask your doctor to show you a graph of cancer statistics dating back to 1955, not just from 1995. Fifty years is more revealing than ten. Or research it on the Internet.

Here's more about cancer from a 2002 flier printed by an endoscopy center:

"As you may know, colorectal cancer is the second leading cause of cancer-related death in the United States. Approximately 160,000 new cases of this disease will be diagnosed in the year 2003, and The National Cancer Institute estimates that more than 56,000 people will die this year alone of colorectal cancer in the United States."

That's over one thousand funerals <u>weekly</u> in 2003. In 1975, cancer incidence was 75 percent higher than in 1933. Diverticular disease of the colon has doubled per capita from 1955 until today. The colon, like the canary, is absolutely warning us of our peril.

"The National Cancer Institute estimates that more than 56,000 people will die this year alone of colorectal cancer in the United States."

Consider too that if you had less bile, excess calcium in the colon might cause hemorrhoids from the strain. And you might feel depressed from a growing load of hard soaps inside your digestive tract. And ovarian cysts may be associated. I mean, what has changed the past fifty or seventy years to knock this country end-over-tea-kettle?

Agree with me on this point -- adequate bile for digestion is key to your health, your ability to be clean inside, your aging process -- and to your beauty.

Here's how Tonya Zavasta puts it: "Our bodies were created in the image of God, the Supreme Beauty. When our actions are in opposition to nature, the results are different types of bodily ills, deformities and ugliness. Since there can be no natural beauty without eating natural food, most of you have never seen the natural you. Beauty lies latent under cushions of retained fluids, deposits of fat, and sick tissues. Your beauty is buried alive, but in most cases it can be revived in a version that will be satisfactory to you. You must take immediate action to revitalize it."

The misleading fiber factor

After reading Adelle Davis, I noticed the following article, which was published in my local daily newspaper. Read it with the fresh understanding of the important role bile plays in digestion, assimilation, and elimination. Note the confusion afflicting experts with the American Cancer Society, Oxford University, and those from around the world.

From what you read in the previous chapter about the true cause of constipation and the limited role fiber would play to improve it, see if you know more than the experts! This is the unedited article published in *The Tennessean*.

Headline: **FIBER MAY NOT WARD OFF CANCER**

LONDON (AP) -- *Evidence is mounting that fiber might not prevent colon cancer after all, with a new study suggesting that one type of supplement might even be bad for the colon.*

The theory that a high-fiber diet wards off the second-leading cancer killer has been around since the 1970s, but the evidence was never strong. The concept began to crumble last year when the first of three major U.S. studies found it had no effect.

In the latest study, published this week in <u>The Lancet</u> medical journal, European researchers found that precancerous growths, or polyps, were slightly more likely to recur in those taking a certain fiber supplement.

The findings demonstrate the difficulty of trying to figure out the relationship between nutrition and disease, said Dr. Michael Thun, who heads epidemiological research for the American Cancer Society.

Fiber is particularly complicated, he said because there are various types and they all could act differently.

"The concept of a healthy diet continues to be the recommendation for overall health," Thun said. "But the painful process of clarifying which ingredients in food do what will take us decades to sort out."

Thun said the American Cancer Society will revisit its recommendations on fiber and colon cancer in light of the growing body of evidence eroding support for the theory that it wards off the disease.

Experts recommend a low fat, high-fiber diet rich in fruits and vegetables and whole grains because it has been shown to reduce the risk of heart disease, high blood pressure, diabetes and some other cancers.

"There is definitely something dietary going on with bowel cancer, but we haven't really been able to fix on what it is," said

Dr. Tim Key, a cancer researcher at Oxford University who was not connected with the study. "The cause of colorectal cancer is very far from understood."

The latest study, conducted by scientists at the University of Bourgogne, France, does not address the effect of a high-fiber diet, but of supplements of one type of fiber -- ispaghula husk, a compound similar to psyllium that is not part of the average diet.

Psyllium, a grain grown in India, is found in some over-the-counter laxatives and fiber supplements.

The study, involving 552 Europeans who previously had precancerous growths in the bowel, found that 29% of those receiving the supplement got at least one new tumor within three years. That compares with 20% of those given fake granules. The findings may or may not be related to the role fiber in general plays in bowel cancer but, considered with other recent studies, the plausibility of a protective role looks less likely.

"This does produce more evidence for the negative side," said Dr. Lesley Walker, a scientist at the London-based Imperial Cancer Research Fund, which was not connected to the research.

"But we still haven't got the totality of the evidence we want," Walker said. "There are still some important ongoing studies under way on the fiber question that should give us some solid answers. Sorting out the influence of genes, food, pollutants, living habits, and other factors requires drawing together information from many different scientific approaches."

The question is, are you willing to wait *decades* for Dr. Thun and Dr. Walker to figure out what is going on with your health? I'm not.

After reading the next few pages, you'll know even more.

It might take two minutes.

Bile impairment from liver poisons

From an edition of my local weekly newspaper, *The Nashville Scene*, comes a story from a syndicated column called "News of the Weird." I quote:

"Trial got under way in January in which residents of Anniston, Ala., are suing for compensation for Monsanto's (and its corporate successor, Solutia Inc.) routinely having dumped deadly PCBs into the ground and local rivers for 15 years after it knew, from the company's own research, that the pollution was so deadly that fish in the rivers died bloody deaths 10 seconds after initial exposure to the water. According to documents from a chemical-safety organization and published in *The Washington Post*, Monsanto and its executives actively hid the dangers from its factory's neighbors while also dumping millions of pounds of PCBs into oozing open-pit landfills. (Monsanto no longer produces chemicals but does make genetically engineered food, which, it assures consumers and the government, is totally safe for human consumption.)"

You now know this much: fiber, constipation, and colon cancer comprise one small corner of contemporary culture. When companies like Monsanto dump PCBs and poisons into streams and rivers and into our homes through our food and water supply, the liver and gall bladder are directly affected. This contributes to an already toxic internal environment and a lack of sufficient bile due to liver exhaustion.

"Fiber, constipation, and colon cancer comprise one small corner of contemporary culture."

As the colon backs up with hard soaps, the liver not only cannot detoxify the blood which circulates throughout the putrative digestive tract, it cannot detoxify *itself* as more vitamins and minerals exit the body. Added vitamin supplements can't be absorbed properly under these conditions either.

Furthermore, natural intestinal bacteria, which are beneficial to health, die, allowing yeast fungus and putrative bacteria to thrive in the digestive tract. These excrete more poisons into your gut. As the negative spiral declines, some seemingly unrelated ill symptom surfaces as medical doctors in white coats march into the picture.

How do they react? By prescribing drugs, which more often than not, also poison the liver. Why? Because the liver naturally filters chemicals from the blood. To get an idea of how a prescription drug feels to the liver, leave a pill on your tongue to dissolve. That bitter chemical taste otherwise goes straight for processing to the liver. Notice also that side effects of pharmaceutical drugs list liver disease as a potential problem.

If the old medical paradigm persists that digestive disorders are from nervous disorders, then a doctor's prescription will likely include one designed to reduce anxiety. Ironically, when you have the feeling like you need to use the bathroom, but can't, that does put an edge on the nerves.

We have been led to believe wrongly that the brain releases chemicals to keep the body in balance, but it is the neural network in the gut which does this job. If ninety-five percent of serotonins, or feel-good chemicals, release from the gut, imagine what happens when the colon gets congested with hard feces resulting from a toxic liver. You're not going to feel very happy.

If this absurd cycle of man-made chemicals poisoning the human body wasn't so tragic, it would be hilarious. Because the executives at companies like Monsanto have all the same doctors as the neighbors they pollute. They're all swallowing the identical pills for nerves, a condition which one way or another stems from serious widespread digestive disorders -- the basic origins of which have been totally missed by the so-called experts.

Our bodies meanwhile are loaded with toxic sludge -- layers of it -- and most doctors deny it is even there.

What *is* the most immediate and necessary first step to end the madness? Clean the colon with water. It is also the most effective aid for freeing the liver to clear itself.

As an added note, you should be aware that Monsanto has been buying up all the seed stocks in America which grow our food. Soon every meal you eat will have Monsanto's thumb print on it. You wouldn't know it, but your liver will.

It also means that natural seeds are being genetically modified to allow farmers to use triple the amount of pesticides on crops. We're looking at over one billion pounds of bug-killer sprayed annually on our food supply. Your individual rate of consumption is somewhere between one and three pounds annually. Factoring in artificial fertilizers and herbicides also saturating the soil, that's a load of chemicals you are ingesting (and your liver is filtering).

Enjoy!

And thanks, Monsanto.

How to increase bile flow

If you suspect that you are deficient in bile, don't panic. Your liver is just as smart as your brain. It knows how to take care of itself.

How will it take care of itself? First, it sends a coded message to the brain that it is in trouble. If translated it sounds like this: "May Day! May Day!" Then the brain tells other parts of the body to pitch in, like the skin and the lymphatic system. The brain gets permission by the general tissues to store chemicals in fat throughout the body. The colon is told to conserve its energy and hang on until the crisis is averted. Then the adrenal system starts pumping high octane's just like it would if your house was on fire.

Your brain also directed you to sit down and read this book. Now that you are here I'll hand the microphone over to your liver. Liver, you've done a great job and we commend you.

"Then the brain tells other parts of the body to pitch in, like the skin and the lymphatic system."

YOUR LIVER: "Hi -- it's an honor to get to speak to you today (your organs are naturally polite, by the way) and I wouldn't be here if it weren't for the efforts of all the organs -- skin, you're awesome ... lymphatics, gotta love ya ... gall bladder, thought we lost you for a second there! Anyway, folks have been asking me what I need and really I think my good friend the colon is in worse shape at this point. As long as he's hurting, ain't no way any of us are getting out alive. I should never be seeing poop up here and I'm telling you I've been seeing poop, not to mention *smelling* it creeping up for years.

Whew! Not to panic, but somebody out there is trying to poison me. At first it was chemicals here and there, your basic pesticides, and then poison's been coming at me like pills and more pills. So somebody has got to shut off the chemicals I'm getting. I tried to pass some of it to Gall Bladder and he starts coughing and sneezing, so I've been storing chemicals in my own tissue and you gotta know that ain't helping me manufacture bile. So everything's out of whack -- cholesterol's all sticky -- and I'm needing oil. Brain's been telling you that oil is bad for the body, but I need it, worse -- I crave it! Then all we're getting are these greasy foods like fries. I need quality oil, like raw flax, sunflower and coconut, not that deep fried vegetable stuff. I'm getting choked up just thinking about it. I've been getting plenty of water, thank you, but the types of chemicals I'm seeing require an *oil* to clean it out. There's two types of toxic chemicals, just like there's two types of paint -- water-based and oil-based. To get the idea of what I'm saying here, you can't clean oil-based paint with water and neither can I clean things up around here when you're only giving me water. Not till I get a quality oil are we seeing much of Bile. And like I said, none of this mess is going anywhere until we get some help with Colon clearing out the pathway ahead. It's going to be some work and take some time, but I know we're up for the task. Thank you, Brain, for this opportunity. Tell Mouth I appreciate the chewing efforts, especially with the salad. That's something else you can do -- eat more green leafy salad -- organic please thank you very much! And we need probiotics down here. Boy do we need probiotics! Don't let me get carried away. Brain, tell me to shut up so this person can get back to reading. Just one more thing -- Heart, I love you, *we* love you. Sorry about all the cholesterol, but you know I'm just doing my job. When I'm back to my old self, we're all going to <u>PARTY</u>!"

Deeper issues of dark circles under the eyes

Meredith came to see me recently for a single session. She is a fifty year-old business owner, prim and professional. She explains: "I am taking handfuls of vitamins and still feel tired all day. Will colon hygiene help me?"

"When was the last time you felt healthy?" I ask.

"I can't remember," she replies laughing with the realization.

I suggest that the first step is to move her to an undeniable feeling of health. "You need a bench mark," I explain. "You can't find more energy when you've forgotten the feeling. Once you feel it, then you can seek to maintain it."

Under Meredith's eyes are dark baggy circles. "Dark circles are a key indicator that your digestive tract is toxic," I say.

She shifts in the chair while explaining that she's had dark circles under her eyes most of her adult life and this was inherited, a family trait. "Uh huh," I say, "We can get rid of them." I suggest that she needs five sessions in a row, once daily if possible.

She takes a deep breath and says, "Okay." Her calendar allows her to finish the five within nine days. Good enough.

My colonic system uses a 5-gallon tank filled with warm water. Positioned two feet above a massage table, the water flows by gravity. The force of water is gentle, but can fill the colon with as much as it will comfortably hold, roughly one to two quarts. Fecal matter in the colon loosens, then purges-out into a rubber tube leading from the rectum to the plumbing system. A clear acrylic section allows for viewing the nature of the release.

"Will colon hygiene help me?"

The goal is to remove as much fecal matter as possible from deep within. The average colon is five feet long and a couple of inches in diameter. The width has been known to swell to nine inches like an overloaded vacuum cleaner bag.

To say that the digestive tract is "tubing" is like saying that a computer is wires. And by comparison, the human gut's construction makes a computer look primitive.

The gut is fully interactive. It provides our most intimate connection to the outer world. Every square inch of the body connects to it down to the smallest hair. The impressive "brain matter" of the gut performs chemistry calculations that modern science barely understands -- conducting them flawlessly day after day and hour after hour.

To catalog the entire process would fill an encyclopedia. "The gut" has memorized every minute detail with provisions to adapt on a moment's notice. The first time the human digestive system encountered a Twinkie, it knew exactly what to do.

If spread flat, the gut's inner surface area could cover a tennis court. Its internal fluids are equally impressive. They flow like a picture-perfect mountain stream cascading through a virgin forest. No joke -- the gut's insides are no less an example of nature's excellence if only hidden from view. Living there are angels, *legions* of tiny angels, who guard and assist us even as we sleep. In lesser terms, these beings are more commonly known as bacteria.

Bacteria have been slandered. Without bacteria, life would cease to exist. I am not referring to the evolution of life. I am referring to *your* life. If the body is the hardware, your health is programmed by the software supplied by the bacteria within. They share their intelligence and protection at no charge -- Nature's share-ware.

When the inner bacteria are abused, the whole body suffers. The best estimation of the quantity living in you: Add-up the total number of individual cells comprising your entire body and the teeming bacteria inside should still outnumber that.

Don't chug a pint of Listerine at the thought. These bacteria are only helpful. You want them there. They are not randomly placed, but like dogs they guard your house. Stephen Jay Gould writes in *Full House*: "Bacteria, by any reasonable criterion, were in the beginning, are now, and ever shall be, the most successful organisms on earth."

How kind they are because they bring their success -- to you!

The human body is so interwoven that a pimple on your face has a connection to "a pimple" in your gut. Dark puffy circles under a person's eyes means that there's similar inflammation in the gut. How can I be so certain? Because colon hygiene eliminates such circles under the eyes, not sometimes, but every time.

The outside mirrors the inside.

I did an Internet search using the words, "dark circles eyes." This led me to several web sites featuring information on the topic. The explanations all stated that dark circles have an unknown cause, probably hereditary, and most likely a natural result of aging and the thinning of the skin around the eyes. More misinformation.

I see people every day with these dark circles.

During roughly one-in-a-hundred colonic sessions, fecal matter in the colon is so backed-up that it creates pressure at the rectum so that fluid escapes around the scope. This creates a nasty mess and a potential embarrassment. This happened to my client, Meredith, the one with dark circles under her eyes. Like a birthing coach I encouraged her to ignore the mess: "Whatever it takes, let's get this stuff out! Keep it coming."

It proved to me that she was in the exact right place. One reason that the condition of the colon affects the eyes is that lymphatic tissue surrounds the eyes. Lymphatic tissue is one of many inner trash-removal systems.

Deeper inside, the colon receives waste from the small intestine and then a valve closes to prevent fecal matter from flowing back. The illeocecal valve can stick open and many doctors have concluded that it is of faulty design. Few have considered that "garbage in" does not automatically transition to "garbage out."

A diet of processed food gums the inner valves. Poisons from fecal matter flushing back into the small intestine are then absorbed into the blood. Under this condition, the liver becomes overloaded. Unable to filter the chronic toxic load, waste is dumped into the lymphatic system for removal -- not the natural course of things.

If the skin thins around the eyes, it does reveal the condition of the lymphatic tissue underneath, inflamed and burdened by poisons. Every bodily system goes into "three-alarm alert" and all available energy is diverted to purge toxins. People with dark circles appear exhausted because they are exhausted -- internally.

Under this condition, the helpful bacterial populations have been wiped out. The entire body is under a stink-attack as the gut literally rots from within. Colon hygiene acts to unplug the sewer. The liver responds by dumping its poisons, as does the lymphatic system. The eyes brighten. As the downward toxic spiral is reversed, friendly intestinal bacteria, or flora, can multiply again and re-populate the digestive tract. They return to displace disease-causing bacteria, yeast, and larger parasites.

The linear progression stated here is simplified, but the bottom line is that colon hygiene removes dark circles from under the eyes. The larger question is why so many Americans now have such dark circles.

For three years I homeschooled my son -- from eighth through the tenth grade. During this same season of my life, I began my professional practice in colon hygiene. As I noticed that some clients would lose their dark circles after several colonic sessions, I coincidentally noticed something shocking.

My son and I watched a video of the 1938 Olympics as a study on pre-war Germany, since it was held in Munich that year. As the camera panned into the crowds I said to my son -- "Those people look *healthy*!" I would rewind crowd shots and could not find a single face with dark circles under the eyes. I watched other old videos and found the same thing.

Following World War II, radical changes in farming began. People's faces from films through the 1950s in America still kept their rosy glow. Starting with James Dean, faces began to change. Elvis acquired puffy dark circles roughly this same period, as did John Wayne. Starting in the 1970s, pale and ghosting actors were captured on film with regularity. Steve McQueen's health fades almost as if his films were time-elapsed.

The statistics tracking cancer mushroomed ten-fold across the twentieth century (1900 to 1999) and it's also recorded right there on our most beloved actor's faces.

Nobody can go to a doctor and get help for dark, puffy circles under the eyes. It's not even considered a bonafied *symptom*. Doctors today think in terms of "pills or surgery" and neither can treat the cause of a telltale condition brewing from within. In fact, pharmaceuticals only contribute to America's poisoned inner landscape. This is one bubble that must burst before cancer statistics run right off the charts.

"Nobody can go to a doctor and get help for dark, puffy circles under the eyes."

With the toughest cases of internal congestion, the darkness under the eyes actually gets worse during colon cleansing before it gets better. I have to be very careful about creating an expectation of an instant beauty treatment. Getting well can be as complex as the causes. As the colon releases poisons, the entire inner-network stirs. In Meredith's case, she did not release a single ounce of poop during the first three tanks. When this occurs, some will suggest that perhaps they are "clean." "Unfortunately, just the opposite," I must clarify: "Your poop is as hard as concrete."

"Yes, I know," is the usual reply.

As the fourth tank of water filled during this first session, here came the rush of internal garbage from Meredith's colon, hard rocks in a flood of orange water.

Later that same afternoon, I bumped into Meredith at the health food store shopping for the supplements I had suggested. "You already look better!" I said. She smiled appreciatively, announcing that others had noticed too. Over the course of sessions she improved 180-degrees in the right direction -- both in feeling and looks.

"Where do I go from here?" she asked me after her final session.

Having recovered a basic feeling of clarity, energy, and wellness, she now had a standard whereby to measure her progress. That put her in the "driver's seat" to follow her own intuition. She had purchased Cape Aloe, an herb which mildly cleans the digestive tract and removes fecal matter. I encouraged her to give herself an enema when feeling sluggish or to return for a colonic if the dark circles returned. Some clients can go months without a major internal flush and maintain clearness around the eyes.

Often I hear the comment: "Won't I become addicted to using water to flush my colon?" The reverse is actually true. A congested colon loses its natural muscle tone.

Lastly, my new client added intestinal flora, also known as probiotics, to her regimen of daily supplements -- those bacteria beneficial to the body -- billions per capsule.

"If you take nothing else," I admonished her like a preacher: "Supplement flora!"

In summary: Colon hygiene improves a person's appearance around their eyes, especially dark circles and puffiness. The reason is because congestion in the colon prevents other organs from dumping toxic waste and requires extra work from all elimination organs including the skin and the lymphatic system. Beneficial bacteria throughout the digestive tract cannot live under these putrid conditions and the body loses bacterial support as well. A toxic person looks like a corpse because so much of the life inside has literally died. Vitality returns as the inner house is cleaned, allowing bacteria to once again thrive and to support health in the ways Nature intended.

If you look in the mirror and see a pale, puffy face staring back, you are a prime candidate for colonics or whatever form of internal hygiene you find agreeable. Visit www.colonicexpert.com to learn more.

The supreme value of intestinal bacteria

You may have read in the news that scientists are concerned that the widespread use of antibiotics by people and farm animals has created resistant strains of bacteria that could bring new epidemics of untreatable diseases, like avian flu and mad cow disease. This threat barely registers in light of the damage antibiotics have *already* done to health in America.

All bacteria are not created equal. The bad ones are in the smallest minority, like terrorists hiding within the heart of a city. Treating a bacterial infection with antibiotics is equivalent to dropping an atomic bomb -- the enemy might be obliterated, yet so with it, everything else is destroyed. Think of pictures of Hiroshima. It's exactly like that.

The miracle of antibiotics has evolved into America's primary health scourge.

In the book, *Antibiotic Crisis: Antibiotic Alternatives*, Leon Chaitow, N.D, D.O., cites a list of diseases associated with damaged bowel bacteria (flora). These include:

- **Acne** -- from a toxic state of the intestines,
- **Allergy conditions** -- from irritated bowel mucosa and the production of histamine, which some types of bacteria produce "when the flora is unbalanced,"
- **Auto-immune diseases** including **rheumatoid arthritis**, Lupus and Ankylosing spondylitis, in which certain "associated bacteria are excessively present,"
- **Bladder infections,**
- **High cholesterol** levels, with "only about 15 percent coming from the diet," writes Chaitow. "Friendly bacteria act to salvage and recycle good cholesterol,"

"The miracle of antibiotics has evolved into America's primary health scourge."

- **Heart disease** -- friendly bacteria protect the entire cardiovascular system,
- **Irritable bowel syndrome**, "commonly associated with bowel flora damage,"
- **Cancer**, potentially triggered by "cancer-forming substances being created in the intestines" if harmful bacteria displace friendly flora,
- **Candida albicans overgrowth**: "Treating the local outbreak of yeast infection without also dealing with what is happening in the bowel will not control the situation for more than a short time," Chaitow explains,
- **Colitis**, a chronic inflammation of the lower bowel,
- **Chronic fatigue syndrome** -- linked to "a weakened state of the normal bowel flora,"
- **Food poisoning**, more likely to occur with a reduction of healthy flora populations (such poisonings estimated at 325,000 hospitalizations annually and 5,000 deaths),
- **Liver diseases**, because good flora help to reduce the "toxic load" in the body,

- **Menopausal problems**, including osteoporosis, since flora bacteria recycle estrogen,
- **Migraine headaches**, triggered by "tyramine," a chemical which negative intestinal bacteria can produce that toxifies the blood,
- **Muscle pains**, including **fibromyalgia**, "directly associated with bowel dysbiosis ... linked to a weakened state of normal bowel flora."

Chaitow notes that "this is only a <u>partial list</u>, since almost all conditions of the human body may feature some aspect of *bowel dysfunction* as an associated factor."

One reason for this -- intestinal flora maintain a healthy condition of the intestinal lining. When populations of flora are killed, the lining becomes chronically weak and damaged. Anti-inflammatory pain killers, including aspirin, block not only pain, but short-circuit the healing mechanism critical to normal bowel function and repair.

A healthy intestinal barrier prevents disease-causing bacteria, fungus, and other potentially toxic substances from entering the bloodstream. When this barrier breaks down, the body then invests energy to fight invaders allowed through, including undigested food particles escaping into the blood. Net result -- exhaustion.

Fungus can grow inside our warm, moist, dark insides, sending roots through the colon wall, not unlike tree roots cracking a sidewalk. More microscopic particles breach the barrier. This produces oxidants to cope with the onslaught, more free radicals that impair a person's overall health.

Seventy percent of the immune system is located within the lining of the digestive tract and intestinal mucus. Elizabeth Lipski, M.S., C.C.N., explains in her book, *Leaky Gut Syndrome*, that this system "provides a line of defense against bacteria, food residue, fungus, parasites and viruses. It neutralizes invaders and prevents them from attaching to membranes." A disruption in proper microbial balance allows other disease-causing bacteria to "wander" to other parts of the body: "For example," Lipski writes, "Blastocystis hominis, a bacteria which can cause GI problems, has been found in the synovial fluid of people with arthritis."

Reviewing the "partial list" of diseases associated with a decline of the intestinal flora, you will find pharmaceutical drugs have been created to treat these same problems. You would expect, at the very least, that antibiotics would be on the short list of pharmaceuticals given to patients. If a common library book can identify diseases stemming from the loss of beneficial microorganisms within the body, certainly you would expect doctors to respect this antibiotic reaction of killing the good flora.

However, exactly the opposite is true. Antibiotic use is at record highs.

After his wife became seriously debilitated after taking a single antibiotic pill, Stephen Fried, an investigative reporter, wrote a book titled, *Bitter Pills -- Inside the Hazardous World of Legal Drugs*. He writes that antibiotics are the second most commonly used drugs in the world and are "improperly prescribed 40 to 50 percent of the time. Either they aren't necessary at all, or the wrong drug, wrong dose or wrong duration is prescribed. Apparently everyone in medicine knows this except the patients."

In my case, I merely had become curious about why my clients were carrying around a huge sack of poorly digested garbage in their guts. The disease statistic which had caught my attention was the dramatic five-fold rise in diverticular disease amongst Americans. Diet certainly was a factor, but so was the discovery of a widespread decimation of friendly populations of intestinal flora from the use of antibiotics; friendly bacteria that otherwise could help to prevent such pockets of infection.

Suddenly, as a new colonic therapist, I was staring in disbelief down the sacred halls of medicine itself as a major contributor to illness. And across the fields of America's farms.

U.S. farmers dump a billion pounds of pesticides over the land each year (causing an estimated 6,000 cases of cancer each year -- but who really knows!? That's about one day's worth of new cancer cases in America). According to *The New York Times*, farmers now use 1.2 gallons of petroleum-based fertilizer to grow a bushel of corn, chemicals which obliterate major sources of friendly microbial bacteria in the soil that otherwise would be a natural food-source of micro-flora supplementation.

"U.S. farmers dump a billion pounds of pesticides over the land each year."

The #1 customer purchasing antibiotics is farmers. The wonder drug for humans has proven to be a wonder drug for farmers because antibiotics fatten farm animals and shorten their time before slaughter. Yet as with people, the cholesterol-lowering benefits of flora are lost on the animal, which has significantly higher saturated fat content in the meat's flesh. Fat also stores chemical residues ingested through the animal's diet.

According to *The New York Times*, feedlot cattle suffer from a weak immune system that makes the cow susceptible to "everything from pneumonia to feedlot polio." More than 13 percent of feedlot cattle have abscessed livers. "As the acids eat away at the rumen wall, bacteria enter the bloodstream and collect in the liver," says *The Times*, "What keeps a feedlot animal healthy -- or healthy enough -- are antibiotics."

Farm-raised fish suffer the same fate. Salmon are kept in pens so crowded that antibiotics are absolutely necessary for their survival. Their gray flesh is dyed pink and their meat possesses none of the beneficial Omega 3 fats of wild salmon.

Just about any farm animal you might eat has been crowded and raised on antibiotics. Eighty-percent of all cattle slaughtered in America have grown fat at one of the five major national feedlots. The pastoral cow eating grass has been sacrificed to the 99-cent burger. Most cows you see on farms are on the path to a feedlot.

Fried wrote in *Bitter Pills* that the estimated profit margin of the nation's drug companies in the early 1990s was about $2 billion per year. $9 billion was spent on research and another $10 billion on marketing.

More is spent on creating demand for drugs than on research. Perhaps that's the good news. The bad news is that pharmaceutical corporations control medical research. They've invested in medical schools, training new doctors, and provide most all the seminars that established doctors attend. The focus on illness is all about pills, pills, and more pills. The latest and the greatest.

Americans pay fifty percent more than Europeans and about a third more than Canadians for the identical drugs. The prediction is that drug costs will bankrupt Medicare. And donations going to cancer research is another form of robbing the poor to give to the rich. Do pharmaceutical giants really need our nickels and dimes to conduct research so that they can then make zillions in profits? Seriously -- how long have we had "walks for cancer" and who benefits from the collecting of the proceeds?

Should it really require *years* of research to explain why cancer was rare just two generations ago? This crisis refuses to be solved with the invention of a pill. I wonder if perhaps the line graph of cancer growth these past fifty years mirrors the growth of the pharmaceutical industry ... up, up, and more up.

Meanwhile, drug profits trickle down as donations to the campaigns of those in both political parties. Candidates then run on a platform which includes "more drugs for seniors," really just the visible tip of an iceberg. But no matter what your age, marketing dollars have pinned you somewhere on the legal drug map. Depression was not on the short-list of illnesses caused by a lack of intestinal flora, but it ranks near the top. If the drug(s) you take requires a *daily* dose from now till death, then a marketing department has driven the invention of your pill, not health care. (Just a rule of thumb.)

Prevention magazine informs its readers that two year olds should check their cholesterol levels. Obviously adolescents are the new target for cholesterol-lowering drugs. Market saturation of those 40-plus is the reason. Intestinal flora have provided that same cholesterol-lowering service naturally (and freely) for thousands of years, but antibiotics have conveniently killed them off.

Hence the demand for new designer drugs.

What's next? A relatively obscure magazine called *Adbusters* has seen the future. It explains: "Novartis, the maker of both Gerber baby food and the stimulant drug Ritalin, with sales over $30 billion and operations in some 140 countries ... looks to a 'simpler' future, when Gerber babies don't have to mature into Ritalin toddlers, but rather can receive their drugs -- and a complex blend of other 'body basics' and 'health stabilizers' -- in a single dietary source. Nature's perfection."

Unless somebody has a better suggestion, why not?

From the back of the room, I expect you to raise your hand with questions. This includes those folks with dark circles under their eyes who recognize that the ghost of death has begun to show through. This includes those who realize that virtually everything which passes through their mouth serves to suppress beneficial bacteria in their gut. This includes those who can recognize that as the "software" of the flora is re-populated, the "hard drive" of physical health re-boots.

We have now touched upon some of the diseases associated with a lack of beneficial bacteria or "flora". What are some of the benefits they provide?

According to Elizabeth Lipski in her book, *Leaky Gut Syndrome*, these include:

- Flora play an important role in our ability to fight infectious diseases, providing a front line in our immune defense.
- They manufacture antibiotics, acids and hydrogen peroxide which makes the intestinal environment hostile to competing microbes.
- Some types of flora provide anticancer and antitumor properties.
- Friendly flora also manufacture many vitamins, including the B-complex vitamins biotin, thiamin (B1), riboflavin (B2), niacin (B3), panthothenic acid (B5), pyridoxine (B6), cobalamine (B12) and folic acid, plus vitamin A and vitamin K.
- Lactic acid-secreting acidophilus and bifidus increase the bioavailability of minerals which require acid for absorption: **calcium**, copper, iron, magnesium and manganese.

According to Leon Chaitow in *Antibiotic Crisis: Antibiotic Alternatives*, intestinal flora help to:

- Improve the body's ability to digest milk products by producing the enzyme lactase,
- Aid digestive function overall and improve the body's ability to absorb nutrients from food,
- Speed bowel transit time,

- Prevent amine formation (ammonia) and other cancer causing chemicals from forming internally,
- Decrease levels of cholesterol in the system, reducing dangers to the entire circulatory system,
- Assist in recycling estrogen, which helps overall hormone balance as well as reducing overall menopausal symptoms.

Simply stated, Lipski explains that "these bacteria live in a mutually beneficial relationship that has evolved to enhance our health and theirs. We offer them a warm, moist home with lots of food, and they, in turn, provide vitamins and other substances that lower our risk of disease and cancer."

Intestinal flora also prevent constipation and foul gas. One way they accomplish this is through one final contribution -- they die. The accumulation of billions of dead bacteria inside the intestines creates a slippery stool. In a body teeming with flora, up to one third of the stool can be composed of those dearly departed bacterial cells. Primitive cultures did not require toilet paper because their stool slipped out in a gel-like casing.

While the cause of constipation is generally misunderstood, the treatment of it is totally wrong-headed.

Bernard Jensen, D.C., Ph.D., the father of colon hygiene, wrote with great detail and insight into this condition. In his book, *Tissue Cleansing Through Bowel Management*, Dr. Jensen writes: "Constipation is a serious menace to health and vitality ... The consequences of this common but subtle malady are becoming more and more prevalent in our society. It is a root cause for many troubles in the body. It is also a symptom of a larger picture that many doctors haven't taken into consideration as yet."

"While the cause of constipation is generally misunderstood, the treatment of it is totally wrong-headed."

Those words were written almost a quarter of a century ago and the contributing factors for constipation have only gotten worse.

The primary question always remains -- "Do you want to be well?" If so, taking the necessary steps will be up to you. That is, create an internal environment that is friendly to populations of beneficial bacteria. Check with your local health food store for supplements which provide these bacteria for your body.

Two roads diverge in a wood; the one "less traveled" leads back into the original and more-primal nature of things. The more-traveled road leads folks to their local hospital.

Take your pick.

Do not become "a water out of fish."

If you enjoy the sport of fishing, then you appreciate that fish live in all different sorts of waters. A fish found in a Florida swamp usually cannot live in a Minnesota lake. What thrives in a Montana creek would never survive in the Mississippi river. Ocean fish caught at the equator look nothing like fish from Alaskan waters.

You can't remove one type of fish from its natural habitat and assume that it will transplant to another type of water, say from a river to a pond or from an ocean to a lake.

However, some fish *can* be transplanted from one water source to another and an avid fisherman will tell you that a trash fish can spoil a lake or river. Or a change in temperature or algae growth can also spoil fishing prospects.

In other words, fish require a specific balance of factors to live. When America was first settled, waters everywhere were teeming with life stemming from eons of natural balance. The foundations of growth began with tiny microscopic organisms which fueled the food chain and remain to this day.

The human body functions similarly. Within it are zones which support unique creatures, namely bacterial forms such as acidophilus and bifidus. When a person takes an antibiotic, the entire inner landscape is transformed. This then changes the balance of life which populates the digestive tract. In the analogy to fishing, an antibiotic kills all the sport fish and sets up conditions for junk fish to thrive. And it supports algae growth which prevents the sport fish from ever returning.

"When a person takes an antibiotic, the entire inner landscape is transformed."

Many female clients seeking colon cleansing tell me that they are trapped in a negative cycle of yeast infections, then bladder infections, then antibiotics, then more yeast, then depression. This has persisted for so long that they forget they did not have these problems before they first took an antibiotic at some point years prior.

Beneficial bacteria living inside the body manufacture hydrogen peroxide which serves to keep the digestive tract naturally sterile. When antibiotics kill these good bacteria, the digestive tract no longer flows with hydrogen peroxide. In the absence of it, fungus can grow on the inside of the gut just like algae overgrowth. Once that balance has been thrown, a yeast-form produces its own chemical byproducts which serve to prevent beneficial bacteria from competing. Yeast overgrowth then stinks like dead fish!

You could supplement beneficial bacteria all day long while poisons from fungus will kill it before it can take hold and reproduce. The result is a septic colon. In this environment, harmful bacteria thrive, causing infections to organs such as the bladder or the colon in the form of diverticula. Pain sends the person to the doctor, who then prescribes more antibiotics. The same cycle happens with children and ear infections.

Many medicines serve to suppress beneficial bacteria and support yeast overgrowth and future infections. Eventually, more damage and more rotting occurs as digestion becomes fermentation with severe bloating and feelings of depression.

Ask any fisherman how algae can spoil a pond. That pond represents the waters within your digestive system. If you take care of it, it will reward you.

Otherwise, you're like a water out of fish. You'll need to flush out the muck inside and start over. Flushing out muck is the job of the colonic. Then you can populate the waters of the gut with flora to support the balance of life again as Nature intended.

Chapter Three
My career resume and the background report

You may be wondering, "How does one become a colon hygienist?" The answer is -- by pure accident.

I was raised in the Midwest and never quite knew what I would do for a career. My mother told me not to do what my father did, which was owning a commercial refrigeration business. One of my grandfathers encouraged me not to do what he did, which was owning a court reporting business. This gave me a generally negative impression of business and when I went to college, I was drawn to study philosophy with no career goal in mind.

Every journey starts with an inspiration and mine came after I attended a church service held in a barn. We sat on bales of hay. The minister told funny stories about his goats and I was hooked. When people would ask me of my plans following college I told them I was going to seminary. I joined a group of students preparing for seminary who met for supper once a month and I did not fit in at all.

Real growth on the journey begins with a crisis. Mine began when I realized that I knew less after four years of college than when I began. Forget seminary. After graduation my older brother invited me to visit him and his wife stationed with the Coast Guard on Kodiak Island, Alaska. I basically stayed in Alaska for nine years. I worked two years running a printing press and seven years at *The Anchorage Daily News* in the classified advertising department in sales. I got married. My wife was a musician and this eventually moved us to Nashville for her career.

"Real growth on the journey begins with a crisis."

My career went into the toilet and I don't mean colonics. I suppose I was in a mid-life crisis at age 32. I hated newspaper advertising. I expected that my wife's career as a songwriter would save me, but really I was passing through an immaturity, a rebellion, a tantrum, during which I delivered pizza for two and a half years. In some ways the rush of the job and the challenge of being under-employed served me well. And I had always loved pizza, which I ate each and every day.

Overlay this with a health concern I had. Before moving to Nashville, I thought I had a hemorrhoid. Sometimes it bled and I went to the doctor. He checked it out with a smirk and said it was nothing to be concerned over, to eat more fiber. I give myself some credit here because having a hemorrhoid and being told to eat fiber at age 30 told me something wasn't right with my world -- just an underlying suspicion. Yet I was so completely-wrongly informed that I believed pizza was a good source of fiber.

After moving to Nashville, we received a direct mail advertisement for colon cleansing and we tried it, my wife and I, and it wasn't something I wanted to do much of. In fact, I thought it unnatural and potentially harmful then, putting water inside the colon.

Back to my career, I was hired by a Christian publisher to be their magazine marketing director, plucked from the hell of pizza delivery, a miracle really. It seemed to utilize all my skills and my education and I vowed I would never leave. Four years later, the situation had become intolerable. Not only that, but my marriage was in serious trouble. My father told me that he couldn't think of another person with more tragedy than me. Just when you think you are rising like some kind of phoenix from the ashes of life, a giant foot comes down and squashes all hope with a giant thud.

Picture a man cast out from his family, cast out from his job, no car, no money, nothing. That was me somewhere in the year 1996.

I saw a poster for a class on massage therapy and I went -- really on a dare to myself. Afterwards I talked to one of the girls in the class who had a thriving gardening business. She asked me if I would work for her for eight dollars an hour. I met her the next day at a garden, which she told me to weed. I remember she left and I stood there silently in the garden with the sun on my face and my feet in the soil feeling total bliss.

From there I attended massage school and became licensed a year later. I had come a long way from the idea of seminary, from philosophy, from Alaska, from any conception of a life I could have imagined for myself.

Here's what happened next -- my back hurt. Now I am pushing forty and feeling older than my grandmother at age ninety. I even asked her once if she ever experienced chronic back pain and she calmly replied, no. It was killing me. Every morning I woke to greet the day it felt like a red hot poker was jammed into my lower spine.

I could barely crawl out of bed without some serious moaning and groaning. I went to three different chiropractors and at least a dozen massage therapists. I was told my sacrum had an extra vertebrae, my ankles were misaligned, my back muscles were tight, and I was told I had worries stuck in my lower chakra. Nothing helped.

I even tried giving up. That didn't help either.

Finally, as I worked on clients as a massage therapist, I observed that the people with the most pain had the worst negativity. I read a book about the powers of creative visualization and encouraged my clients to become positive thinkers. Then, in a flash of epiphany that had taken my entire life to be sparked, I realized that I had failed to practice this myself.

The first problem I tackled was my low back pain. I visualized myself well, jumping from bed in the morning pain-free.

This power is what led me into colonics. Colon cleansing flew at me fast and furious once I pictured myself well. Like I said, it came about through pure accident. Perhaps I should also mention that it cured my back pain.

Did I say cure? Yes -- *cured* it! Right out of left field. From a positive part of my imagination of which I had no conscious awareness whatsoever. When you get to that realm, nothing comes by accident.

How it began

This book grew out of a visit to my parent's home in South Carolina where they transplanted from the Midwest five years ago. Their success has been to retire well and they deserve it because they worked diligently many years.

Their beautiful home sits surrounded by tall pines, embellished with flowers they've planted by hand. They compost their own fertilizer. A stone's throw from their property is a huge recreational lake on which they sail a splendid sailboat and along the shore they may stroll around a picture-perfect, lighted walking path at a moment's inspiration. Of course, it's safe 24/7 because it's all within a gated community where the guards smile and wave as you leave, even if you're just crossing the highway to the country club for Sunday brunch or for a game of golf.

And they are avid golfers; my father sometimes leads local tournaments and my mother displays a plaque on the wall for hitting a hole-in-one. There's rarely an idle moment. When home, they attend a square dance gathering most every Friday night.

Punctuating their calendar are road trips they take in their monster RV the size of a Greyhound bus. They've maintained life-long friendships all over the country.

During winter they spend at least a month in Florida where my sister lives raising five children. Within the last year they've traveled to Greece and also flew to China and Tibet for several weeks of touring. Then they're leaving soon to sail with my older brother somewhere in the Caribbean. He's a doctor. My younger brother works for a Chicago bank after receiving his MBA from the Kellogg business school at Northwestern University where he graduated with a 4.0 grade point average.

My parents deserve to be proud. They have twelve healthy, happy grandchildren including two from my marriage. Dad served his country as a pilot in the Air Force and Mom served her time as a Cub Scout den mother and Girl Scout leader. My parents were childhood sweethearts and have been together through almost fifty years of marriage which has been a model of sensible partnership.

Somewhere along the way, my path diverged from theirs. Namely, I became a professional colon hygienist. This launched me on a path quite extraordinary from that of the average person and even that of most health therapists.

It is with a great measure of audacity that I should consider I could surpass my mother's wisdom on any subject. Yet -- I have.

This became apparent after my recent visit. My father was out of town when I drove with my kids to visit my mother in South Carolina. We arrived late in the night, so I greeted her in the morning as she was setting pills out on the counter. "What are those?" I asked her. Blood pressure medicine, synthetic thyroid hormones, a multi-vitamin, a baby aspirin, and a tablet of brewers yeast.

I made a suggestion: "Vitamins and pharmaceuticals should be taken separately since drugs can impair vitamin absorption."

She nodded as she took them one-by-one. "Next time I'll do that," she said.

I opened her drawer crammed full of various supplements. "Mom," I said taking them out and reading the labels, "Most of these bottles need to be trashed." She groaned.

"Some of these expiration dates are years old," I explained.

Well, she said she hated to throw anything away. She had a bottle of wheat grass powder five years old. "Your multi-vitamins are no good either," I said.

"I just bought those," she contended.

They were a dime store brand called *Daily Impact for Seniors*. The vitamin E was dl-Alpha Tocopheryl, a synthetic. If the manufacturer cut corners on the E, then you could assume that the rest of the product was mostly packaging and possibly even toxic to the organic human system. Such stuff won't even compost.

"If you place a value on your health," I said to her, "Why would you scrimp on it? This 'shark cartilage' supplement expired nine months ago."

"I'm sure it's still good for you," she replied.

"Mom, it's *fish* ... old unrefrigerated fish!"

She proceeded to tell me that the most difficult thing about living in a retirement community was that one-by-one the people around them were being diagnosed with terrible diseases. A wonderful neighbor has just passed away from colon cancer who was otherwise vibrant and in her prime.

"That's the very reason why you need to nix the aspirin," I said. Even though the stomach might handle the effect of a baby aspirin, over time aspirin weakens the protective intestinal lining. The intestinal lining is extensive and nobody wants this delicate area leaking toxins into the blood stream. In other words, there are side effects, although many presume aspirin is God's miracle pill.

A while later we went to brunch at the country club. The buffet spread included mostly proteins: omelets with bacon and sausage; seafood including salmon, Mako shark, and King crab legs. A server wearing a tall white chef's hat stood waiting to carve slices from a huge roast beef. The vegetables were cooked till soggy, yet were no longer hot.

I perused the salad bar. Here we had plain iceberg lettuce with the standard side additions (like egg salad, potato salad, and macaroni salad) and the usual five dressings loaded with salt, sugar, and partially-hydrogenated oils. It wasn't that I felt ungrateful to be foraging there, fully-aware that many people are starving in the world; however, this was me conducting an informal study of what retired Americans eat at a Sunday brunch.

As my teenaged daughter cruised the dessert bar and scooped up some blueberry cobbler, I overheard my mother comment that she was glad to see her choose fruit with her meal because it was "the healthy choice." This book was born in that moment as I realized most everything my mother taught me about health was wrong. Because adding fruit and sugar to a big protein meal wreaks havoc on digestion, inducing fermentation, supports yeast fungus growth, which forms gas, bloating and much more.

I had explained this to my daughter, and she chose to keep the cobbler, which I encouraged her to enjoy, as I too loved dessert at her age.

Still, I realized that much of what my mom taught me about health, despite her best of intentions, was totally outdated. Each generation discovers these faults, like my grandfather's generation, which consumed eggs, butter, and gravies right to the grave. The generation before that did not understand sanitation's role in preventing disease, and before that, the "bleeding of sickness" was practiced, which likely led to the demise of the Father of our Country,

George Washington, who was bled just prior to his death.

Fast-forward to the invention of the Twinkie and the Big Mac. The problem with these concoctions has less to do with fat grams and obesity; everything to do with stopping-up digestion. Today's civilized colon is so congested that even FIBER has been shown to contribute to precancerous growths. "This does produce more evidence for the negative side," said Dr. Lesley Walker, a scientist at the London-based Imperial Cancer Research Fund, quoted on the topic of taking fiber for preventing colon cancer.

The next revelation of the generations will be that most of our food is poison -- not when it's chewed, not when it's churning in the stomach, but when it passes from the stomach into the twenty-five foot length of intestines where it won't budge.

But don't take my word for it. Visit any local retirement center, sit down for a meal and see for yourself the prize America has to offer its golden-agers. Pay attention, because unless you retire to a grass hut on a deserted island, hard-won success may mock you with cafeteria food and servers who resent seeing your face for minimum wage.

"Today's civilized colon is so congested that even FIBER has been shown to contribute to precancerous growths."

The generation born during the Depression-era are the first Americans to both benefit from and now suffer from advancements: in pharmaceuticals (taking multiple prescriptions), electromagnetic devices (microwaves and cell phones), petro-chemical bug-killers, petro-fertilizers, antibiotic/hormone-laden corn-fed beef, mercury fillings, nuclear energy, margarines, saccharins ... and then corporate mismanagement of precious investments ... stress ... retiring with a measure of prosperity for breakfast in a buffet hall ... all passion worn thin, just the sound of chewing and swallowing, chewing and swallowing ... and you know they think you don't know that none of it moves on its own.

This I do know, that I myself am feeling better than ever at age 47 and feel compelled to share the good news. There is still time to change course -- a small window overlooking contradictions in what it takes to be well today.

So I'm talking about a revolution where real health is possible. It begins with awareness. And unlike previous revolutions, this time, Mom, you're invited.

Mom said, "Have some dessert."

Theories abound regarding health and diet and mostly they induce guilt and frustration. If you're dead-set on having pie with your meal, by all means, have pie. If you enjoy it piled high with ice cream, by all mean, pile it on.

I myself wouldn't do it, but that's just me.

There are as many health concerns out there as cracks in the sidewalk. The reality is that until you understand and grasp any principle, it's still "out there," just something "they" say about where not to tread. The smorgasbord of diet opinions are too many to mention whether you're considering becoming a vegetarian, a raw food fanatic, following Atkins on low-carb consciousness, or anything in-between.

Whatever you decide, bless your own choices. If you're eating pie, then bless your pie!

My mother introduced the concept of food combining to me years ago. However, I observed that she didn't follow those principles and so neither did I. Nobody I ever met gave two hoots about what was tossed together into that iron chamber known as the stomach. No matter what went in, it all seemed to come out poop.

When I turned thirty, I experienced my first symptom of aging: a hemorrhoid. Sometimes it bled, sometimes it itched, and this was quite disturbing. I had heard of a relative who had surgery to remove hemorrhoids and this was not a fate I desired.

Possessing health insurance at that time, I went to my doctor. He checked it out with a bit of a smirk. His diagnosis -- nothing to worry about. He said I had just one and it appeared to be small. His prescription -- eat more fiber.

I had little clue as to what fiber was (and he didn't volunteer any). Eating bran cereal and stewed prunes seemed old-generation. My idea was to snack on raw celery. This lasted about one week. About then I read an advertisement of a new laser treatment for hemorrhoids and figured if my condition progressed, I'd have high tech medicine ream me a new baby-fresh sphincter in the future.

I did try one particular home remedy. My mother-in-law had had hemorrhoids. Her treatment was to take cayenne pepper orally and then stick a capsule of goldenseal herb up her rectum. The story went that one day she got her pills mixed up and accidentally stuck the cayenne pepper up the wrong end and nearly landed in the hospital. After hearing of this I tested inserting a goldenseal capsule and the resulting rectal itching was so bad I thought I'd go insane.

After moving to Nashville, Tennessee, I received a direct mail packet of coupons in our mail box. Flipping through, a two-for-one offer from a local colon hygienist jumped out. Possibly I could flush out the cause of my hemorrhoid from the inside and not only that, I loved getting anything at a discount. I picked up the phone, made an appointment, and coincidentally also changed the entire direction of my life.

The colon hygienist, Lee, shed light on a dark subject. I had always imagined that digestion took place in the stomach and after that, food was converted into feces that wound its way through the intestines on its inevitable path to the toilet. The digestive disorder of which I *was* aware was ulcers, which were supposedly caused by worry. Drinking milk with your meal was supposedly the solution for that, which I often did. Or if one had heartburn, one took an antacid, but I myself never experienced heartburn. I figured, therefore, my digestion was optimal.

I also assumed that the large intestine connected to the stomach, because the food mash dumping from the stomach would be at its greatest volume, then little by little it would be squeezed into poo-matter by the time it reached the anus. However, Lee explained that the colon, or large intestinal plumbing, attaches at the anus, and that its approximate five feet is considered to be an external organ and therefore is perfectly safe to cleanse with water.

For several reasons already discussed, the typical North American colon gets gummed up and won't emit properly which causes a person to strain at the toilet, which puts pressure on the sphincter muscles, and boom -- you have a hemorrhoid. She said that mucus is produced by the body to protect the colon, but this was intended as an occasional need and our modern diets have caused excess mucus to become a daily occurrence. As a person ages, this mucus permanently lines the colon with what she termed "a toxic sock." If someone does enough colonics, they eventually loosen this mucus sock until one day it begins to make a dramatic exit.

Parasites in the colon are also common. She said that she sees them come flowing out of her clients occasionally -- like black earth worms. (I myself have not witnessed these.) Some have tape worms and the way she said to get rid of them is to starve them on a fast and then sit your butt over a pan of warm milk and honey and the hungry thing will slide out into the pan.

I took this shocking information to heart, going on an immediate fast.

"Parasites in the colon are also common."

Lee said that tape worms hated pumpkin seeds so I went on a pumpkin seed fast, swallowing also capsules of cayenne and goldenseal. After two days I felt very sick. But before ending my fast, I squatted over a pan of milk, and to my disappointment, no worm slid out. I phoned Lee, telling her of my ill condition and she had me come right over for a free colonic to flush the cayenne and goldenseal from my system.

Lee sat me down for a heart to heart chat. "Forget about worms," she admonished. Because I wasn't able to afford frequent colonics at sixty bucks a pop, she encouraged me to use herbs to cleanse my system, showing me a product called Intestinal Tune-Up. It contained black walnut hull to remove worms, psyllium and flax seed meal for bulk fiber, cascara sagrada for better elimination, and several other cleansing herbs which were mild on the digestive system.

She told me to get an enema bag from the drug store and to use it as the poor man's colonic. A colonic tank holds five gallons of water which is filled at least three times during a session, which compares to an enema bag which holds a quart or two. A colonic reaches into the entire colon, while an enema just draws out what's right there.

"Won't I become dependent on enemas?" I asked her.

"If your colon was healthy, you might have some concern," she explained. "But the goal is to start things moving, so don't worry about it for now." She stated her optimism that I would continue colonics again soon, so for the meantime to keep cleansing no matter what.

The Tune-Up immediately began removing translucent strings of mucus which appeared floating in the toilet like creepy yellow lettuce. The Tune-Up also made me emit foul gas, which no matter how hard I tried to hold back, still eked out. I think I became immune to my own emissions until one day I overheard a co-worker tell somebody, "It smells like dinosaur farts around here."

I became terrified I'd be publicly discovered. Leaving the common area bathroom after my nasty dumps, I acted non-chalant, but my grin surely betrayed that I was the cat who was swallowing the rotten canary.

I had to ask myself -- was it worth it? I thought maybe not. I quit the whole messy business.

A few years passed and after leaving the corporate scene I found myself in massage school. (That's another story.) When I showed up at one of my classes on hydrotherapy treatments I discovered that our guest speaker was my colon hydrotherapist. She began by announcing to the class that "Scott had done colonics," to which I beamed proudly. After the class, several people asked me about it and I assured them it was something worth doing once.

A few more years passed and I got it into my mind that I should go see Lee for a single colonic session to "clean me up." I had long since quit the Tune-Up and was feeling generally toxic.

Back in her office after seven years, what struck me was Lee's radiance and energy. I had feared that her frequent colonics would one day be the death of her -- that they were somehow not natural and potentially damaging. But she looked so great I commented that she probably still "got carded" and in fact, she told me she had been asked for her I.D. recently by a waiter. Little did he know she was newly a grandmother!

We had a friendly chat during my colonic and then I went on my merry way. My one hemorrhoid rarely bothered me and so I didn't give internal cleansing another thought.

A month later, Lee phoned me. She explained that she had a client who wanted training in administering colonics and needed a partner. Was I interested? She reminded me of the benefits and I half-heartedly agreed to meet together to discuss it. I worked now full time as a massage therapist for a local day spa and was doing quite well. As I reflected on how I would incorporate colonics into my practice, I couldn't imagine it. And my children were horrified at the idea of telling their friends what their father did. So I phoned back to decline.

Our conversation swung me around so that I changed my mind again to try it.

Very significant to this was a seemingly unrelated factor. I had observed that many of my massage clients stressed themselves out by their own fearful thoughts. A book about creative visualization had impressed me and I encouraged my clients to "think away" their stressful situations. "Focus on positive images and desires," I would say, "because thoughts have an expanding quality."

Ironically, my own back had bothered me at the same time I began massage school. I had enlisted all my teachers and fellow students to work their magic on my lower back. Every morning it pained me with a dull ache. I saw chiropractors too and nothing seemed to help. At the time Lee phoned I had just put into practice my own creative visualization -- of me waking in the morning able to bend pain-free.

My partner in colonics training, Chelsea, was a twenty-four year old nurse, a vegetarian, and completely enthusiastic about the benefits of colonics. We began working on each other as part of our study of colon hygiene. The volume of internal junk material which flowed out from both of us was amazing. After we became certified, Lee offered her office to us for a nominal fee and soon we had performed twenty colonics on each other.

During one of these sessions I mentioned to Chelsea that sometimes "my butt itched." She suggested, "It's probably yeast." I went to our local health food store and was amazed at the number of books on the subject of yeast. I bought two books about it.

I learned that our bodies naturally have bacteria which thrive in the digestive tract called 'friendly flora'. The best description I've read about flora comes from a booklet titled "Leaky Gut Syndrome" by Elizabeth Lipski, M.S., C.C.N. She writes:

"Does it surprise you to know that there are more bacteria in your digestive system than cells in you body? Four pounds! ... The proper balance of these microbes is essential to the health of our digestive tract and total body. They manufacture antibiotics, acids and hydrogen peroxide which makes the intestinal environment hostile to competing microbes."

Imagine food landing in the digestive tract like Dorothy arriving in the Land of Oz. Friendly flora are like the Munchkins who point the way on the yellow brick road. Munchkins are happy and kind and also vulnerable. If the wicked witch takes control over Oz, guess who's going to greet Dorothy upon her arrival? Evil winged monkeys.

Yeast is an evil winged monkey in the digestive tract. If yeast gets an upper hand, your future health is at stake. How so? Because yeast fungus doesn't facilitate digestion, but fermentation and putrefaction. This means gas, malabsorption, increased intestinal permeability to toxins, skin problems, premature aging, and a whole list of clinical conditions you don't want.

Eighty percent of the bacteria inside the body should be of the beneficial kind. This keeps the negative effects of "bad" bacteria and yeast fungi at bay.

Fermented mash doesn't pass through the twenty feet of small intestine and the five feet of large intestine according to natural design. This trips the first domino on a downward spiral. There hasn't been much medical research about the negative effects of yeast and increased intestinal permeability, possibly because the remedy is one of prevention and not cure, which is more the playing field of alternative medicine. Much has been written about it, but who really wants to curl up with a book titled "Leaky Gut Syndrome"?

And anyone can think of at least one person who eats worse than they do, who is doing just fine, which means we all believe we are "healthier than average." Meanwhile, one hundred years ago, only one person in thirty died from cancer. Today, cancer kills almost one in three Americans and will afflict four out of five during their lifetime.

Diverticulitis has steadily grown over the past century from affecting ten percent of the U.S. population over age forty-five now to half. This condition means that the natural pockets of the colon have become impacted and swollen. It's a civilized disease because in primitive cultures, diverticulitis is unheard of.

Cancer is killing Americans off like a terrorist attack of the September 11th magnitude occurring every two days *all year long*. Line up who's still healthy and half of those over age 45 have swollen pockets of rotten, yeast-infested garbage crammed in their colons like crackers and pus stuffing a mouth that desperately needs to whistle.

"Diverticulitis has steadily grown over the past century from affecting ten percent of the U.S. population over age forty-five now to half."

Bernard Jensen, a twentieth century pioneer in the field of colon hygiene, studied many stool samples of average Americans and found nearly all with an exact inverse ratio of bad bacteria to good: eighty percent bad to twenty percent good. This means that as a general population we've been feeding our yeast and not our friendly flora. What feeds yeast? Fiberless products made from processed white flour, drinks made with yeast like beer and wine, most dairy products and sugar.

Two centuries ago, Americans consumed about 15 pounds of sugar annually. When the Civil War broke out, that consumption had nearly tripled. Then it doubled again at the turn of the last century to 85 pounds and from then till now it has increased again to where every year we nearly consume our own weight in sugar. For now, forget that refined sugar is translated by the body into sticky fats and cholesterol. Forget that cardiovascular disease was rare two centuries ago and has risen in similar proportion to our intake of sugar.

Sugar feeds yeast. Yeast then sets up a dictatorship in the digestive tract, subjugating friendly flora.

The book "The Yeast Syndrome" defines it like this: "The yeast syndrome is actually an old disease that has become newly predominant in industrialized Western nations largely arising from 'high tech' alteration of external environments and the resulting assault on the internal body environments ... Large numbers of people show signs and symptoms that have them functioning at very low levels of wellness ... If left untreated, C. albicans wreaks havoc throughout the human system."

For me, my symptom was that I had minor itches, sometimes in my ears, which was not bad enough to raise flags. The body continually makes subtle corrections toward wellness which pass below the threshold of awareness. If this corrective process deteriorates, some obvious symptom will manifest. A symptom signals that some conscious action may be required to bring the system back into balance.

One of my options was to treat my occasional itching topically with a cream or a suppository. Another option was to explore what was behind the itching, to better understand my body. One is the path of resignation; the latter, proactivity.

Proactivity tackle puzzles. Solutions can be complete surprises.

Through exploring the possibility I had yeast fermenting my insides, I discovered that there were natural products which can help counteract the effects of yeast proliferation, namely caprylic acid and grapefruit seed extract. One of these products was called *Yeast Cleanse*, which I took immediately.

My surprise was the discovery that **my lower back pain and my itches were connected.** The next morning I woke to my amazement that the *Yeast Cleanse* helped eliminate my lower back pain instantly -- even if temporarily.

At this time I worked part time as a massage therapist in a chiropractor's office. Many of the patients came every week with the complaint of lower back pain. They returned again and again with minimal improvement. I explained to the chiropractor that low back pain might be of digestive origin because mine had vanished after taking a product which helped reduce yeast. He listened briefly, asked no questions, and went about his work as usual. I thought possibly he didn't grasp what I was saying, but I shut my mouth for the sake of keeping my job.

My low back pain did return, but at half its usual intensity. My pain also seemed to rise and fall according to the pattern of my internal cleansing, often dropping down to zero after each colonic.

When Chelsea and I reached forty colonics together, we both experienced other remarkable changes. Hers came when she said she felt intense pressure in her abdomen during the colonic and needed to get down from the table. She went into the bathroom and gave birth to a monster which she insisted I come look at. The rotting smell was so intense that I grabbed a towel to cover my nose. Floating in the toilet was something from a horror movie -- a gruesome mask with a twisted expression. What I saw was like half cow pie, half raw liver, intertwined in a mass equaling about a quart.

We gawked speechless at each other as she flushed it down.

I hadn't noticed that Chelsea's complexion prior to that was yellow, something I figured was hereditary, a sallow tone. After she had dropped that wretched load, the next time I saw her, her complexion was pink and bright, like a different person. Everybody who knew her noticed this change -- she radiated.

I also passed something startling at this time. After my colonic, I too sat on the toilet and passed demons. As water passed out it burned like fire. The ammonia stench was so powerful I needed a towel again over my nose. The water was otherwise clear, but I can't tell you the relief I felt flushing the toilet. Lee explained that the poison released was likely from a pocket of parasites which gave off ammonia from their negative metabolism. The practical result was that my lower back pain lessened again permanently to about twenty-percent of the original intensity.

Over the years I've been a patient of about ten chiropractors and worked as a massage therapist for two. Their training includes four years of college and another three or four in chiropractic school and they see most dysfunction as originating at the spine. Pain to them means subluxation of nerves. Open the nerve path and out goes the pain.

The chiropractor I work for is diligent and caring, but he showed no interest that the digestive tract has an equal number of nerve endings as the spine. He ignores the disease statistics which point to diet as the major American subluxation of general health. He made no time to investigate how I personally and significantly reduced my chronic low back pain through creative visualization, anti-yeast supplements, and colonics. Why? None of that relates to his spinal study and also, it's not good for repeat business.

Can you imagine most chiropractors sitting down with a patient for creative visualization -- "Now I want you to imagine yourself living completely without back pain."? Not very likely! There are exceptions, certainly.

The division between medical doctors (the A.M.A.), chiropractors, licensed massage therapists, and colon hygienists is regulated and specific. However, how *you* approach your own health isn't regulated. Therefore, your own investigations and conclusions become as meaningful and unique as you are as an individual. One single learning can trigger all sorts of realizations.

For example, I picked up a book by best-selling health author in the 1970s, Adelle Davis, called "Let's Get Well." In a chapter on digestion she writes:

"Antibiotics taken by mouth kill the (good) intestinal bacteria, thus causing severe vitamin K deficiencies which often result in internal hemorrhages, and deficiencies of folic acid and many other B vitamins. Conversely, when attempts have been made to produce vitamin B6 deficiencies in volunteers, a few showed no signs of a deficiency for an entire year, presumably because the vitamin was amply supplied by the (good) intestinal bacteria. ... Therefore, *health can depend on the amount of vitamins produced in the intestines.* The growth of these valuable bacteria also depends on the general diet. (Parenthesis and italics mine.)

Gas distention indicates that putrefactive bacteria are being fed rather than one's own body. When putrefactive bacteria are allowed to grow, they produce histamine, causing allergies, and liberate quantities of *ammonia*, which irritate the delicate intestinal membranes, pass into the blood, ... and cause other manifestations of toxicity. In many disease conditions, the toxicity from ammonia from this source imposes serious health problems."

My point here is to chart how my awareness of my body (itching and a hemorrhoid) started me on a direction that may have saved my life, not to mention dramatically improved the quality of health I now enjoy. These minor symptoms uncovered my problem with yeast, which meant I was deficient in crucial cancer-fighting B vitamins made by flora, and facilitated the discovery of ammonia in my intestines.

Doctor's records will show that I underwent a complete physical exam just prior to these discoveries and I was given a clean bill of health, yet I was far from healthy. Because I don't have health insurance, it was my mother who coaxed me to have a medical exam, and even paid for it. I appreciated her thoughtfulness, and obviously she's supportive of my own findings that went beyond the scope of my doctor's assessment.

The surprise benefit was the discovery that my low back pain was not related to my spine, and my chiropractor never would have correlated back pain to a yeast problem. Despite all the progress that's been made in modern and alternative medicine, guess what? You are on your own! To stay healthy you must become your own best health detective.

In fact, I'm certain that my yeast problem originated during my teen years from *medicine*. When I developed pimples back then, our family doctor prescribed the antibiotic tetracycline, which I took off and on daily for years. Many of my friends used it and their mothers endorsed it, same as mine. According to Adelle Davis, tetracycline given to young children was found to cause "unsightly yellow pigmentation" on their teeth, thought to be from the destruction of vitamin E. She goes on to say that "a number of drugs interfere with digestion and the absorption of all foodstuffs and of most vitamins and minerals, resulting in deficiencies which, in turn, cause some damage to every part of the body."

Truthfully, I'm grateful and lucky to have survived to my forties without a major malady.

B vitamins produced by proper intestinal flora not only feed the body, but the mind. In his book, "How to Live Longer and Feel Better," Nobel prize-winning author Linus Pauling writes: "The fact that a deficiency in the intake of vitamin B3 leads to the mental illness associated with pellagra caused me to check the medical literature. I found that persons with a deficiency in vitamin B12 usually become psychotic even before they become anemic. Mental disturbances, I found, are also associated with deficiencies of vitamin C (depression), vitamin B1 (depression), vitamin B6 (convulsions), folic acid, and biotin, and there is evidence that mental function and behavior are also affected by changes in the amounts in the brain of any of a number of other substances that are normally present."

Now when you see TV commercials for medicines which help specific symptoms, perk up your ears at the end when they start listing off potential side effects and know those are just the *beginning*. No wonder that sales of anti-depressants are soaring as a bizarre side effect of the other medicines we take which impair vitamin absorption.

"When you see TV commercials for medicines which help specific symptoms, perk up your ears."

Now that I've bashed some of what's typical of American lifestyle, allow me to finish where I began -- dessert. What's more American than apple pie?

You may be anticipating that my conclusion is that dessert is made from sugar and sugar feeds internal yeast fungus, so avoid dessert. Not necessarily so. What you eat or drink is merely one factor of digestion. What you eat *together* complicates matters most.

I end this section by quoting from a little book first published in 1951 called "Food Combining Made Easy," written by Herbert M.

Shelton. It's been reprinted at least 31 times. Read what he has to say and then draw your own conclusions on pie eating.

"A few years ago I sat with a group in the home of a friend and viewed a television program. On one of the commercials a cereal bowl was placed before us on the viewing screen. Before our eyes a huckster poured the bowl full of a popular breakfast food. Into this, he dumped two heaping teaspoonfuls of white sugar. Over this he sliced a banana and poured onto the mixture he had created, a handful of raisins. Finally, he poured over the whole mixture a liberal quantity of milk or cream, which was sure to have been pasteurized. As he demonstrated the preparation of the breakfast dish, he kept up a running fire of words intended to convince the television audience that the mixture of food he had put together was both tasty and nutritious.

No animal in nature ever eats such a haphazard comminglement of heterogeneity. It does not speak well for human intelligence that millions of men, women, and children, continue to eat such meals day after day and take drugs to palliate the resulting discomforts.

All sugars -- commercial sugars, syrups, sweet fruits, honey, etc., -- have an inhibiting effect upon the secretion of gastric juice and upon the motility of the stomach. This fact adds significance to the remark made to children by mothers that the eating of cookies before meals 'spoils the appetite.' Sugars taken with protein hinder protein digestion.

Sugars undergo no digestion in the mouth and stomach. They are digested in the intestine. If taken alone they are not held in the stomach long, but are quickly sent into the intestine. When eaten with other foods, either proteins or starches, they are held up in the stomach for a prolonged period, awaiting the digestion of the other foods. While thus awaiting the completion of protein or starch digestion they undergo fermentation.
Based on these simple facts of digestion, our rule is: Eat sugars and proteins at separate meals."

THREE SIMPLE THINGS YOU CAN DO
STARTING TODAY FOR DIGESTION:

- After a meal, wait at least one hour before having dessert.
- Following that same logic, you wouldn't eat pancakes in the same meal with eggs, nor would you wash down breakfast by chugging orange juice.
- Take a supplement of a multi-strain of intestinal flora every day which can be purchased at any health food store. Store in the refrigerator.

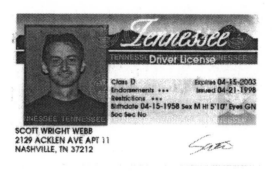

Copy of author's license with photo taken April 21, 1998. Note dark circles under the eyes.

Mom said, "Dark circles mean you need a nap."

Once you grasp a corner of the truth about health (that you know that you know you know), it becomes a cornerstone upon which you can build and continue to revise. A new reality starts coming through which you can see and feel and makes you wonder, "How was I so blind before?"

National Public Radio announced an international conference being held concerning pollution in the planet's oceans. The angle on the news was that this meeting was being held in Des Moines, Iowa, far from the nearest ocean shore. The reason is because farming across America's bread basket uses cheap nitrogen-based fertilizers which run off into the streams and rivers, particularly the Mississippi river, which exits into the Gulf of Mexico. Vast dead spots in the sea have formed which support no marine life. Obviously this is of great concern to those monitoring our oceans, serious enough that they are eager to sit down to chat with the nation's farming community who grow, of all simple things, our *food*.

I raised social concerns with my health mentor, Lee, and the response was always the same: "Clean your colon." For the time being, that was the most socially responsible activity I could perform, to get well myself.

I decided to go into the colon hydrotherapy business after seeing what a tremendous difference it made for me and my training partner. Finding an office to hang our shingle wasn't easy. We required one room with an attached bath where we could tap the colonics system into the existing plumbing. I phoned dozens of potential property managers and once they heard about the nature of our plans, the conversations ended.

But they always had to hear it twice -- "You're doing *what*?"

Finally I persuaded a building owner to concede. He had declined leasing to us until I offered to pay him more rent.

"I decided to go into the colon hydrotherapy business after seeing what a tremendous difference it made for me and my training partner."

Chelsea worked full time as a nurse and is a single parent. Because we were having so much fun with colonics, carving out a couple of hours a few times a week was no problem. After fifty sessions together, my desire for cleansing outstripped her availability. Our new office was located across the street from my home making it more convenient for me.

I decided to administer a colonic on myself, which is how Lee cleansed herself. Here's how the procedure works. You lay on a massage table. The colonics unit sits in a cabinet against the wall raised nineteen inches above the table. Filtered tap water flows into an ordinary five gallon jug from which is attached a rubber hose. The hose connects to a specially designed stainless steel scope which inserts into the rectum about the length of a bottle cork -- not very far, but not particularly pleasant either. The water is driven by gravity into the colon with enough force to enter the body, yet remains gentle. Attaching at the other end of the scope is another rubber tube into which fecal matter flows back out of the body and directly into the sewer system.

Whoever invented the system was a genius. The flow is entirely self-contained -- no odor, no leakage, no problems.

The main challenge working a professional system by yourself is that you must operate the water control with your foot while using one hand to steady yourself on the table and the other to squeeze and release the outflow hose to regulate the internal water pressure. Two pillows prop you up so you can see what exits through a clear acrylic section of the outflow tubing -- the interesting part.

The first time I hooked myself up to the unit, both pillows fell to the floor, as did the clamp on the inflow tube. While controlling the water handle to fill the tank, my foot cramped in a painful spasm. Then the inflow hose came disconnected at the scope and water spurted everywhere. I concluded that giving myself a colonic was not possible.

However, Chelsea had to cancel our next appointment and I found myself right back in the saddle. The second time was a charm and I've not had any trouble since.

Lee said that she could feel fecal matter collecting in her colon. I had never experienced any awareness of feelings in my colon except for the normal call of nature. My regularity was that I usually went "number two" first thing every morning.

After that, why think about it?

To facilitate internal cleansing, I began taking one capsule of a non-addictive herb called Cape Aloe leaf. In the morning I pooped as usual and then in the afternoon I began feeling heavy and sluggish. Even my brain seemed foggy. If I did a colonic, all of that vanished as I would release fecal matter in pieces from one to six inches long totaling two or three feet. I found that if I did four tanks of water I continued to release more and my intuition often pushed me to five tanks. I would feel intestinal pressure during the last tank and suddenly intensely orange water would flood the hose mixed with black sediment resembling pea gravel. The resulting clarity and relief never failed to astonish me.

The school where Lee had trained stated that to fully clean the colon it took fifteen colonics per year of life. If I didn't own a unit I would have scoffed at the idea. It seemed like a ploy for repeat business because there's always going to be something passing in the digestive system. At 43 years old that meant I needed 645 colonics to get clean, a commercial value of about $30,000.

Yet here I was doing a colonic almost daily, up to a hundred total, and I knew I needed more. The difference I felt before and after a colonic was like night and day. Before I had one, the world seemed overcast; then afterward, bright and sunny. I reminded myself of Clark Kent using a colonic booth to transform into Superman.

The nature of my releases changed. Instead of orange and black, the matter coming out turned pale and creamy, the consistency of macaroni and cheese. Sometimes the water would have white webbing floating out as large as my hand. Then I'd feel intense pressure as the whole tube would fill with the stuff. Sometimes I had to continue to almost six tanks because my colon wouldn't stop releasing.

I'm not alone in this. Nearly all my clients can attest to the fact that at some point they release so much volume that from the scope to the wall, the five feet of tubing completely crams full with the release. One client released a gusher of chocolate-colored water that lasted a full four minutes. We just looked at each other in disbelief as it rushed out. Very few considered themselves generally constipated, including me.

Another client comes to see me from Manhattan where she's employed as a teacher and can't afford the $100 fee for colonics there. She practices yoga, jogs about sixty miles per week, eats healthy, and despite the fact that she's 26, feels chronically sluggish.

As I write this, she is visiting her family in Nashville and has come to see me every day. Yesterday was her fourth colonic in a row and the previous three passed no less than four feet of rock-like fecal matter. The dark lines under her eyes vanished after the first day and we've come to take it for granted that each time she leaves my office feeling like a million bucks.

But yesterday was different. She released her four feet of junk almost immediately in one continuous rush. I could feel it rattle the tubing it was so hard. And then nothing, just clear water for thirty minutes. She said she could feel something moving inside and the tubing would sometimes jump like her colon would emit another load, but we saw nothing. So we stopped the session. She went into the bathroom.

After a few minutes she shouted from the bathroom: "Come in here!" As I opened the door she explained, "I exploded."

The stuff in the toilet looked like black paint. It had not the slightest tint of brown or any color tone. "Have you eaten anything different?" I asked her as she stumbled over to a chair to sit down.

"No," she replied, "Just give me a minute to recover."

So I watched her come to herself like something birthed from a cocoon under time-elapsed photography. Finally she rolled her head around in a circle, then fixed her eyes on me and said, "*Wow!*"

I had her stand and take a few steps. I asked her, "Do your hips feel like they're rolling on greased ball bearings?" "Yes!" she replied.

"I love that feeling," I said as we joined in the same club of getting out the inner blackness and feeling totally, incredibly awesome. Before she left we jumped around and danced together.

Constipation must be newly defined or surely it will redefine us. We must awaken to the fact that we are living under a bizarre twenty-first century health paradigm.

Constipation is not as simple as the National Digestive Diseases Information Clearinghouse defines it -- "the passage of small amounts of hard dry bowel movements, usually less than three times a week." *Consistency* and *frequency* are outdated concepts.

I repeat, consistency and frequency are basically meaningless today.

The best opinion on constipation I've heard is from someone who's been practicing colonics for fifteen years. When I first asked her about it she shook her head and muttered under her breath what I imagined are obscenities. That says it all. Asking her about what to take for constipation is like asking an avid downhill skier what sort of wood makes the best skis. We're on a whole different mountain slope than we were just thirty, forty years ago.

"Constipation must be newly defined or surely it will redefine us."

I came across a brochure at a health food store titled, "STOP: Constipation is a serious health concern." It states that "the natural medical community" has a specific belief about regularity, that "it is healthiest to have three bowel movements per day nearly every day."

"Unfortunately," it says, "most people have only one bowel movement or less per day."

This brochure then builds a case against constipation which can be alleviated by taking certain products. Under the headline, "**The Constipation Solution: The 30 Day Advanced Cleanse System,**" it states: "Unfortunately, the problem with constipation builds up slowly over time, and takes time to improve when not supported by a specific program for success ... Eventually, I began to formulate what I considered to be the most effective program for achieving 2 to 3 gentle bowel movements per day and for improving the overall condition of the colon."

I applaud the resourcefulness, but I guarantee you that taking herbal products till I was age-ninety would not have dislodged the gallons of foul "macaroni and cheese" that erupted from my colon after one hundred colonics. The goal of 2 to 3 "gentle bowel movements" per day misses the mark of the truly radical action required today to clean the colon.

Don't be suckered by huckster-talk.

It would be wonderful to believe that there somewhere existed a "natural medical community," if each weren't a contradiction of terms. Anything "medical" falls under the jurisdiction of the A.M.A. and they are very touchy about their turf, which includes all disease. Anything "natural" is whatever doctors can't prescribe and drug companies can't synthesize and patent. "Natural" is something found in nature which supports health and the prevention of impaired health.

And there is no common "community" among natural health practitioners like we're all wearing tye-died T-shirts holding hands and singing around a camp fire.

If you think about it, each expert merely represents the various fields and modalities of a health concept at least partially bogus. Constipation receives little attention from medicine *or* natural modalities. The "health" businesses that thrive off it make laxative products which fly off the shelves of grocery and drug stores. The customers who buy bulk fiber at those same outlets do themselves a great disservice.

"Experts" say that one third of what's solid in a stool should be made up of bacterial flora, which are lactic-acid organisms that displace gas and odor-forming bacteria and fungus such as yeast. The fiber of fresh fruit and vegetables is important mainly because it supports an environment of healthy flora, *which in turn help to form proper stools*. When the friendly flora are depleted, fiber alone can worsen the problem of constipation. That's because the typical American bowel is so gummed up with toxic material, fiber can't pass through. It's like throwing big rocks down a chimney to remove a blockage.

Some folks are having frequent bowel movements, but the fecal matter is passing through a channel lined with more fecal matter. If they think regularity is a sign of good health, they are most deceived.

One of my massage clients has suffered from fibromyalgia -- feeling muscle soreness every minute of the day. The quality of her flesh is the most alien I have ever touched, like Styrofoam. I offered her a free colonic treatment knowing she would experience instant and tremendous relief. Her complaint included that she had a bowel movement but a few times per week. "I wish I was like my late husband," she expressed several times, "After every meal he would excuse himself to use the bathroom."

Figuring that they had been married many years, sharing a similar diet, and that he had died from a terrible disease, I finally suggested that he might have been just as backed-up as she.

"He may have been using the toilet *frequently* because his stool was passing though a colon packed with fecal matter," I speculated. "In that case it would have been pencil thin."

"Pencil thin," she replied. "Yes, it *was* pencil thin."

For whatever reason, this client could not bear the thought that fecal matter might be poisoning her internally or have a connection to her fibromyalgia. She never has taken advantage of my offer for a free colonic.

Sadly, most of the customers buying bulk fiber are also taking a plethora of medicines, which in turn kills healthy intestinal flora, which then supports the fallacy of adding fiber supplements. If this weren't happening, half the U.S. population over age 45 wouldn't have diverticulitis or diverticulosis, which is a ballooning of the colon with excess fecal matter and mucus.

One expert in the "natural medical community" certainly is Andrew Weil, M.D. In his best-selling book, "Spontaneous Healing," digestive disorders are given merely two pages out of 375 total. His assessment is that mostly they are stress related and the recommended diet modification is to eliminate coffee, tobacco, and alcohol. He writes, "A common root cause of many digestive disorders, from esophageal reflux to constipation, is an imbalance between the intrinsic motility of the gastrointestinal musculature and the regulating influence of involuntary nerves that coordinate the whole system. There is so much nervous input to the GI tract that it is very susceptible to stress-induced distortions. In fact, along with the skin, the digestive system is the most common site of expression of stress related illness."

For as cutting edge as Andrew Weil's information has been, for me, it suddenly became old school. His assessment sounded as if taken straight from a medical textbook. I see he has a new book out about aging, but I haven't had time to look it over.

Author Adelle Davis, in her book "Let's Get Well," suggests another possible internal condition connected to constipation (and it's not nerves!). Hard stools can result from a poorly functioning liver and gall bladder and this is nothing to be taken lightly. She writes:

"The gall bladder, a pear-shaped sack hanging between the lobes of the liver, is a reservoir for bile. When food containing fat leaves the stomach, hormones cause the gall bladder to empty by inducing vigorous contractions in its muscular walls and simultaneously stimulate the liver to produce more bile at an accelerated rate.

Although bile contains only water, lecithin, cholesterol, minerals, acids, and pigments, it is vital to health. Its lecithin content breaks down fats into microscopic droplets that can be readily surrounded by enzymes, digested, and absorbed; and its bile acids are essential before digested fats, carotene, and vitamins A, D, E, and K can be carried across the intestinal wall into the blood.

When a diet is low in protein or high in refined carbohydrates, little bile can be produced. If the amount of bile is insufficient ... fats remain in such large particles that enzymes cannot combine readily with them; hence fat digestion is incomplete and fat absorption markedly reduced.

Part of the undigested fat quickly combines with any calcium and iron in the food to form insoluble soaps; thus these minerals are prevented from reaching the blood, and the hard soaps, causing overly firm stools, bring about constipation."

It should be plain that a high-fiber diet would do nothing to improve constipation resulting from a poorly functioning liver and gall bladder. Both of these organs can become inflamed by the use of drugs or from toxic chemicals in the environment including common pesticides, and from bacterial and fungal toxins such as those from Candida yeast. When "Let's Get Well" was published in 1965, our environment was just beginning its toxic descent, despite the beginnings of environmental control groups at that time.

Regardless, fiber without <u>sufficient</u> intestinal flora present is a senseless supplement. Even though we've gone to the moon and beyond, something so simple still baffles scientific medical researchers at the turn of this new millennium.

The dark circles under my eyes, which I've had for years, my mother assumed meant I needed a good nap. Raising two children and supporting my family has often required compromising my sleep. I figured she was right. Naps are great.

Over the past year, however, I've replaced nap time with forty-five minutes here and there on the colonics table.

One Saturday I went to my office to mop the floor. I had done *five* colonics on myself over the previous three days. The reason for so many was because it felt like something significant was moving itself down. Every one of those five colonics released great volumes of material.

While in my office I debated with myself whether to do another colonic. I wondered if possibly I was becoming obsessed with internal cleansing. The little devil on my shoulder told me I was, but the little angel convinced me to jump up and do one tank "just as an experiment."

In the first five seconds, brown hunks began flowing out. One tank led to two, which led to three, then four, then five. Literally every time I put water into my colon, something of substance flowed back out like a regular chocolate bar factory. After forty minutes I began calculating the length of matter which had so far passed out from my body.

I wanted to be conservative, so I based my time on thirty minutes. Conservatively also, I figured I released two inches of fecal matter every thirty seconds, but I released actually about every twenty seconds. End to end, my total release was at least ten feet long. Even if I somehow exaggerated, let's say I released eight feet or only six feet.

I am five foot, ten inches tall and have weighed one hundred fifty-five pounds for years. Where was I storing all that trash? Let's not forget that this was my sixth colonic in three days, all of which were super filthy, even after months of regular colonics.

I finally climbed off the table and felt like I had never felt in my entire life, like shackles and a ball and chain fell free. I immediately got on the telephone and called anybody and everybody whom I thought would care.

"I just released ten feet of shit," I screamed over the phone, like I'd won the lottery. When I phoned my mother, she asked me "what I had been eating," as if I was somehow unique and other people didn't also possess such internal trash.

A few colonics later, I used the toilet to release any excess water from my bowels. A small white, square object floated innocently on the water and it struck me as odd that just one kernel of corn would have come out. As I reached to flush, it dawned on me that I hadn't eaten corn.

Fishing it out, I brought it to another colon hygienist, asking, "Is that what I think it is?"

"Yep, it's a section of tape worm," she confirmed.

"How sure are you?" I asked. Her reply was to laugh.

"I'm thinking of going to the doctor to get some poison," I said.

"Don't you dare!" she said seriously. "But, do whatever ..."

I hated the thought that I had a tape worm gorging itself inside. Makes you want to commit hara-kiri right there on the spot just to get to it.

I didn't go to the doctor. Remember, I had just been to one for a complete physical exam and was given a clean bill of health. But I can't blame my doctor. Tape worms are asymptotic and unless you go into it knowing what to look for, you'll never find it. If I thought I might have had a symptom, it was a little twitch I got sometimes in my side which I thought was a tiny muscle spasm.

My other symptom -- dark circles.

Tape worms don't cause dark circles under the eyes. The environment in which they thrive may. Natural intestinal flora manufacture hydrogen peroxide and other beneficial substances that keep larger parasites out. So taking a prescriptive poison systemically is an unnatural disaster to the body. Because if your flora population is weak, and you take a poison to kill worms, flora are wiped-out too. In this poisoned internal environment, yeast fungi thrive, which welcomes bigger parasites right back.

Having a tape worm meant my body wasn't able to keep it out. But my body was undergoing radical change and began to fight back as it detoxed, as evidenced by that one section of the tape worm dislodging. Knowing I had released ten feet of fecal matter meant that this volume of poop had otherwise been locked inside my body either in length or stuffed into a ballooned section of my colon. Losing that was key.

Connecting the small intestine to the large intestine is an important valve called the Illeocecal valve. After digested matter enters the colon, this valve is intended to close to prevent that same matter from washing back.

"Dark puffy circles around the eyes are from excess particles of fecal fluids that have nowhere else to exit."

Tape worms can attach themselves to the small intestine and then hang down. If one were to grow past the Illeocecal valve, the valve might not fully close. And if fecal matter is backed up, it might not close regardless. Some doctors today believe that the valve is of faulty design because many people have valves which don't close properly. However, diet plays a major role in gumming the Illeocecal valve; and it is the American diet for which we weren't designed, not a defect in the valve itself.

If the Illeocecal valve remains open, toxins flowing back into the small intestine are picked up into the blood stream and lymphatic fluids. These toxins then need to escape somehow because if the valve is clogged enough to get stuck, the liver isn't faring much better and can't filter the blood well. Dark puffy circles around the eyes are from excess particles of fecal fluids that have nowhere else to exit. If you take a nap, the rest the body receives helps it to cope somewhat, but is only of slight cosmetic benefit. The slightest stress and they come right back till dark circles become a permanent feature.

At the day spa where I worked as a massage therapist, the aestheticians gave me an eye cream designed to reduce puffiness. But it's merely a topical solution for deeper issues literally brewing from within.

The best remedy for dark circles: **clean the colon.**

The best remedy for a toxic liver: **clean the colon.**

The best remedy for constipation: **clean the colon.**

For tape worms: **clean the colon** -- plus use elbow grease, as I will explain.

The other colon hygienist suggested that I take powdered barley greens because the enzymes in it irritates the protective shell around the head and body and colonics can then loosen its grip. She also said it could take several months up to a year to lose a stubborn tape worm.

I went to our local health food store and poured through the book section like it was a library, looking up "tape worm" in the indexes. I wrote down all the herbs listed by various authors that would help dislodge my unwanted friend. My goal was to inform it that it had worn out its welcome!

I went to the bulk herbal section of the store and selected various powders including garlic, onion, clove, goldenseal, cayenne, and oregano. I made my own capsules. I bought another product called "Rascal," made by the Kroeger herb company.

Over the next couple months I consumed pumpkin seeds, raw onion and garlic, and cucumber sprinkled with sesame seeds, sometimes collectively making up an entire meal. I spoke to the tape worm too, telling it to get the hell out.

Over the next month I also bought and consumed three bottles of an enzyme product called "Purify," made by Enzymedica, Inc. It contains pharmaceutical grade protease derived from plant sources. Their brochure explains how it works:

"It is known that proteases are able to dissolve almost all proteins as long as they are not components of living cells. Normal living cells are protected against lysis by the inhibitor mechanism. Parasites, fungal forms, and bacteria are protein. Viruses are cell parasites consisting of nucleic acids covered by a protein film. Enzymes break down undigested protein, cellular debris, and toxins in the blood, sparing the immune system this task. The immune system can then concentrate its full action on the bacterial, viral or parasitic invasion."

Sometimes I would go to my office at night for a colonic to possibly catch Mr. Worm off-guard. I watched the tubing very closely for any signs that he decided it was time to leave. Two months passed.

One morning, the first object to exit my body during the colonic was a rope-like section of mucus roughly ten inches long folded over three times. As I sat up, it passed out of the tube, but another section of similar size passed right behind it. Then came a third, which I carefully observed to be composed in square sections.

Was that my worm?

Not long ago I underwent bioenergenic testing by a local therapist, Nancy. Her unique software and computer-driven machinery can read the life-force of nearly every bodily system and give it a reading on a scale from one to a hundred. A score of fifty indicates that the tested system is balanced. A lower score indicates restricted function and a score over fifty indicates over-function. It works similarly to how a lie-detector machine reads energetic and nervous impulses.

One of my concerns was that my frequent colonics were depleting my electrolyte balance and my intestinal flora. Colonics have also been suspected to deplete vital minerals such as calcium, magnesium, and potassium.

I sat quietly in a chair as the testing began. Not long into our session, Nancy began saying "Wow!" a lot.

"What's going on?" I asked her.

"This is remarkable," she replied.

"What?"

"Your systems are perfectly balanced."

Her software produced a graph of all my readings, which all ranged between a score of 48 and 52, mostly dead-on 50s. "Extremely rare," she said randomly pulling up another client's chart to show me what's typical. The twenty or so readings bounced erratically between the low 40s to the mid-60s.

Nancy's machinery can also pinpoint exact vibrations of parasites by type.

"What about a tape worm?" I asked her.

"Nope," she said re-testing for that specifically, "It's not coming up."

"Well, bless him then for leaving," I thought to myself.

I phoned my hygienist friend to tell her of my results. I told her, "Nancy seemed amazed that my systems are balanced across the board, even my electrolytes."

My friend replied, "I test the same way. One of these days people are going to grasp that colonics help the body to completely balance itself. How can the body be in balance when it's jammed full of poop?"

The real test came during this last visit with my mother. As we were saying goodbye, she said, "You look good, Scott."

I can now proudly say, "Look Maw, no dark circles!"

THREE SIMPLE THINGS YOU CAN DO FOR DARK BAGS UNDER THE EYES:

- Clean the colon with herbs:

Take "Aloes" (Cape Aloe Leaf).

"Intestinal Tune-Up" may be purchased at many health food stores. It is manufactured by Honeycombs Industries, Montrose, Colorado.

Health food stores offer many brands of colon cleansing products and they all work differently for different people. Experiment, but avoid products with psyllium as the main ingredient.

- Clean the colon with water:

A series of three to 15 colonics gets the process started. Consult the yellow pages, other health practitioners, or the Internet for referrals. If funds are tight, purchase an enema bag from a drug store and give yourself an enema, especially helpful when combined with taking colon cleansing herbs. I can't tell you not to obsess on cleaning, just don't obsess.

- Eat whatever you want.

I heard the story of a preacher who told a drunkard that if he became a Christian, he could drink all the whiskey he wanted. The man embraced Christianity and then returned to the preacher saying, "You tricked me! You knew I wouldn't want alcohol after becoming a Christian." The preacher laughed and said, "I told you that you'd drink all the whiskey 'you wanted.'"

The same principle applies to diet: Consider your colon and eat whatever *you want*.

Chapter Four
Corporate advertising budgets also buy public relations

One client phoned to tell me about an excellent Oprah Winfrey show in which two doctors brought real human colons. One colon was healthy, the other ballooned and distorted. Later that same day, another client told me that I had missed this awesome show, but I could see parts of it online at Oprah's web site.

First thing when I got home, I pulled up that show. The "Aftershow" did not feature the two colons. It highlighted the audience asking questions of the doctors. A lady asked if a person's colon was misshapen and distorted, was there a way to correct that? The doctor replied to take baby aspirin. Not one, but *two* every day. He lectured on and on about the benefits of baby aspirin which registered off the scale of my horror meter.

"Whoa!" I thought, "That was some *bad* information." I wrote an email to The Oprah Winfrey Show that two daily baby aspirin would help to CAUSE a diseased colon. Never in a thousand years would aspirin snap back a colon into its natural, healthy shape. Of course my email was lost in the pile, one of thousands the show receives daily.

"I wrote an email to The Oprah Winfrey Show that two daily baby aspirin would help to CAUSE a diseased colon."

I was waiting to get a haircut reading the July, 2005 issue of *Reader's Digest* when I stumbled onto an article by Michael Crowley titled, *"Payola Profs -- For the right price, they'll betray our trust."*

It exposed a public relations firm based in Washington DC that had been writing columns for years in support of the nuclear power industry and paying local professors to sign their names as the authors.

I have read other accounts of this type of grass roots marketing. Hollywood capitalizes on this every day raking in big bucks for product placement. Like the candy, Reese's Pieces, went through the roof in sales after shown in the film, "E.T." And manufacturers of the .44 Magnum handgun couldn't build them fast enough for years following the "Dirty Harry" movies. And on and on and on it goes.

It would require no stretch of the imagination to think that PR firms not only work tirelessly to get their clients on The Oprah Winfrey Show, but capitalize on every second of on-the-air time, selling it, so-to-speak. Not just on Oprah, but on Leno, on Conan, on Letterman, etc. The pharmaceutical industry spends about $10 billion annually on advertising and some of that is earmarked for PR, not just for paid commercials and ads.

In this case, would you doubt that the doctors on Oprah mentioned aspirin as a "wonder drug" as PR payola? Maybe, maybe not. I will explain why the *Readers Digest* article, for me, suddenly explained the huge leap in these doctor's logic and their display of questionable soundness on a show which is otherwise based on integrity of information. Oprah herself might be shocked to learn more.

First, taking a baby aspirin will no more cure a misshapen colon than it will fly you to the moon. You would be hard-pressed to find a *single* gastroenterologist who would agree that baby aspirin has miracle-healing powers for reshaping the colon.

Secondly, aspirin is WIDELY KNOWN to be a COMMON CAUSE of leaky gut syndrome or "increased intestinal permeability." The following quote originates from a Keats Good Health Guide. According to the publisher, these guides "give you the newest and best available information on health topics of major importance, written by leading physicians and other health reporters, researchers and expert reporters." This particular guide is titled, "Leaky Gut Syndrome," written by Elizabeth Lipski, M.S., C.C.N.

She writes: "Nonsteroidal anti-inflammatory drugs (NSAIDS) like **aspirin**, ibuprofen and indomethacin are a common cause of leaky gut syndrome. NSAIDs work by blocking prostaglandins, which are tiny messengers that circulate throughout the body. Some prostaglandins cause healing and repair; others cause pain and inflammation. However, NSAID drugs block all prostaglandins. The pain may be gone, but the healing process is blocked. Since the digestive tract repairs and replaces itself every three to five days, prolonged use of NSAIDs block its repair. GI side effects are **well known**: the lining becomes weak, inflamed and leaky, causing leaky gut syndrome. NSAID use also increases the risk of ulcers of the stomach and duodenum. These drugs also cause bleeding, damage to their mucus membranes of the intestines and GI inflammation. Even **moderate use** of NSAIDs has been shown to increase gut permeability."
(Pgs. 17-18. Bolding is mine.)

The result of taking two baby aspirin a day are anything but healthy for the large and small intestines. There are about 80 recognized autoimmune diseases that can result from the development of a leaky gut; which coincidentally, it is also well known that the gut contains seventy percent of the human immune system. I'll refer you for further study to another resource book titled, "Gut Solutions," by Brenda Watson, N.D. and Leonard Smith, M.D. See pages 153 to 158.

Some of the diseases associated with increased gut permeability, which can be **hastened** by taking two baby aspirin, include rheumatoid arthritis, fibromyalgia, multiple sclerosis, hives, chronic fatigue syndrome, ulcerative colitis, and diabetes. So I think we'll nix the daily aspirin.

Thank you very much trusted doctors who appeared on The Oprah Winfrey Show. We are going to find a five-foot long wet noodle and beat you with it.

One other detail about aspirin therapy: there are many, many medical studies on aspirin which proclaim that it offers a health benefit. And there are many which tell of adverse effects. When a doctor refers to a particular study, dig to uncover who PAID for the study. It would be an interesting project for somebody to track the results of various medical research studies and who bought the results. Medical research is highly political and don't believe for a minute that it doesn't come down to dollars and cents. And don't be surprised if research sponsored by an aspirin maker comes up shiny like copper.

Not Dr. Ruth!

Isabelle is a massage therapist and we've been friends for several years. She came for a colonic session and I told her the story about the doctors recommending two baby aspirin on The Oprah Winfrey Show, mentioning the possibility that they were paid to promote it.

She replied, "That's probably right." Then she told me a story about her recent experience.

Isabelle works at the Hermitage Hotel, the swankiest 5-star hotel in Nashville. The famous sex therapist, Dr. Ruth, came to Nashville to give a free talk to women on the topic of "menopause and sex after age 50" at the Hermitage Hotel. It was open to the public and Isabelle attended. Hey -- free champagne and hors d'oeuvres!

A second doctor, a female gynecologist, also gave a talk. What struck Isabelle was the constant reference to some kind of estrogen cream as the answer to every woman's health issue over age 50.

After the free talk, Dr. Ruth was signing books. A man wearing a suit stood by the table and Isabelle stuck up a conversation with him. Since he was about the only male in the room, she asked him, "So what is your connection to all of this?"

He explained that he was the pharmaceutical representative from the company sponsoring Dr. Ruth's tour, the maker of the estrogen cream (HRT replacement) for women over age 50. Funny, there had been no mention of "a pharmaceutical sponsor."

Now, if that doesn't have you shaking your head, this will. The following is taken from an article I read years ago in a vitamin supplement catalog. I won't reference it because the article was called a "new feature" and after appearing once, it disappeared.

I suspect that the new feature was yanked after pressure on the vitamin dealer by a pharmaceutical's legal department or from the A.M.A. itself. The title of this interview was: "The facts about drug-nutrient depletion."

DOCTOR: "Here's an example for you: the whole issue of hormone replacement therapy (HRT), which is now all over the news. About five years ago I made a statement at one of the big meetings and said that I really don't think that HRT is going to pan out to be what everyone is saying it is to be. And I heard this 'mmmmm' through the audience. I said to them, 'Here's why.'

HRT depletes the body of vitamin B-6. It also depletes the body of magnesium. Now, let's translate that into clinical practice. If you have a depletion of vitamin B-6, your homocysteine level is going to increase. Homocysteine is an amino acid that, if it is elevated in the blood, will increase your risk of heart disease. You need vitamin B-6, vitamin B-12 and folic acid in order to lower your homocysteine level. So if you are depleted of vitamin B-6, immediately your risk of heart disease is going to go up. That's number one. Number two is HRT depletes the body of magnesium. Magnesium has two roles.

The first role of magnesium is in the maintenance of blood pressure and cardiovascular function. The other is in the bones, which is another area HRT was purported to help in. So what does magnesium have to do with the bones? Calcium and magnesium work together; and magnesium, along with vitamin D, helps transport calcium into the bones. So now you have no effect on osteoporosis, which HRT was supposed to help. We've been given this data for a long time, so I said no; it (HRT) is not going to work the way they were saying, unless you replenish the B-6 and magnesium."

QUESTION: "How significant of a problem is drug-nutrient depletion, especially if you think of it in terms of starting with somebody who is possibly deficient and then uses a nutrient-depleting drug?"

DOCTOR: "I can't even begin to describe to you the acceleration of disease and what is happening to the American public."

One of the doctor's quotes is enlarged and highlighted in brackets which reads:

"By the way, magnesium is the number one mineral deficiency in this country. About 75 to 80 percent of the people in this country are deficient in magnesium and that's why we have sleep problems and that's why we have blood pressure and cardiovascular problems."

<u>Translation</u>: If you attended the free seminar featuring Dr. Ruth and did not know that it had been sponsored by a pharmaceutical company and trusted statements made there, and began using an HRT cream, realize that you just increased your risk of serious disease (like blood pressure and cardiovascular problems) from the side-effects of your new medicine. However, one client of mine who is a nurse suggested that the side effects of HRT could be considered minimal compared to the benefit. Two sides of the same coin?

Isabelle also pointed out to me that her gynecologist seems oddly motivated to get her taking antidepressants. Her doctor kept asking her, "Are you sure you aren't depressed?"

"No, I don't think I am depressed," Isabelle replied repeatedly.

Her gynecologist then had her fill-out a questionnaire to determine whether she was indeed depressed. This was ten questions and the possible answer choices were, "Always, sometimes, seldom, never." Isabelle described it as "really basic," and "I answered the questions proving to the doctor I wasn't depressed."

"No, I don't think I am depressed," Isabelle replied repeatedly."

"What did the doctor say?" I asked her.

"She gave me samples of antidepressants to take home anyway."

"Wow!" I said, "You went for a gynecological exam and the main focus was to get you on an antidepressant?"

"Yes."

"Since when are gynecologists experts on depression?" But before she could reply I asked her another question: "Did your doctor give you a second option to taking drugs?"

"No second option," she replied, "Just the free samples."

What was it we were taught to say? Just say *no*.

I regret repeating this concept, but pharmaceutical drugs have known side effects. One way drugs are being sold is through the news media. Another is through talk shows. Another is through celebrity endorsements. Another is through medical doctors. Seek to find out whether any recommended medicine impairs the liver's ability to produce bile. If yes, review my earlier information on bile. Often you find that a drug's side effects slowly stimulates more underlying causes in a spiraling cycle of new symptoms.

Once you realize that medicines have far-reaching side effects, it's easy to spot information about it in the news. On the cover of a publication called "Bottom Line Health" (February, 2005), are tid-bits of "Late-breaking News." Here's part of one titled: **Antibiotic Alert**.

"Patients who combined the antibiotic *erythromycin* with drugs used to treat high blood pressure or other conditions had a fivefold greater risk for cardiac arrest. *Theory*: Some drugs increase the concentration of erythromycin, which can trigger an abnormal, po-tentially fatal, heart rhythm."

Below that piece of news is another release: "The natural pain reliever methylsulfonylmethane (MSM) is a good substitute for the prescription arthritis drug *celecoxib* (Celebrex) and the over-the-counter painkiller *naproxen* (Aleve). New studies report that these medications may increase heart attack and stroke risk. MSM, a natural compound found in green vegetables, does not cause heart problems or damage the stomach. *Caution*: Consult your doctor before using MSM if you take blood thinner."

I'm thinking, why not just eat the green vegetables?

What *does* heal a misshapen colon?

"A healthy bowel requires sufficient water, good nerve tone, good muscle tone, adequate circulation and the right biochemical nutrients in the right amounts. These, however, are not sufficient

to bring health to a dirty, toxic-laden bowel. Cleansing must come first, then tissue rebuilding can take place. This is not an easy task and I don't believe anyone can do a good job in less than a year's time."

Bernard Jensen, D.C, Ph.D., Nutritionist
Author of "Tissue Cleansing Through Bowel Management"

Candy came for a colonic one day every week for almost one year. Sometimes I felt dread before her appointments and I didn't know why because I liked her tremendously. The problem was -- we were hitting a wall.

Even though fifty colonics a year might seem like a lot, it wasn't enough. Candy was in her late fifties and was bothered with symptoms of illness. She ate healthy, was spiritually advanced, exercised, swam, practiced yoga, loved to laugh and had lots of friends and a wonderful husband. But she wasn't transforming.

Candy approached me one day with an idea. Her house didn't have the extra space necessary to install a home colonics unit, so she proposed that I train her and another one of my clients, Susan, to perform colonics on themselves and install a unit in Susan's home. Candy lives outside the city of Nashville, but drove past Susan's house frequently and could increase her internal cleansing with free access to a unit.

This was totally their inspiration and I thought it was an excellent idea.

"Candy was in her late fifties and was bothered with symptoms of illness."

Not long after the system was up and running, I received a phone call from Susan. She said, "Candy is coming over every other day for colonics. Won't she harm herself?" I got a good laugh out of that one.

Sometimes I bump into Candy around town, particularly at our local health food store. Candy has become transformed. Her appearance changed so radically that I asked her if she had any old photos to compare herself to. She did and I posted them in the bathroom at my office with her permission. It turned out that several of my clients knew Candy and one of them commented that he had seen her recently and did not recognize her. "I thought of her as someone not well," he said, "And now she is radiant!"

Before	After
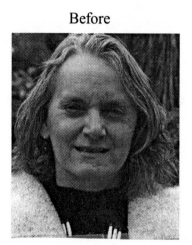	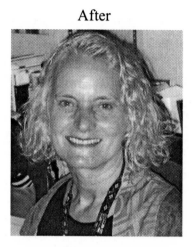

My client, Candy, provided me with her "before and after" pictures. Note darkness around the eyes and puffiness before doing colonics. Some comment that the lighting is different, however, these two pictures illustrate improvements from colonics I see frequently. (Not everyone is willing to put their photo into a book.)

Her determination was so strong to be well that she figured out a way to install a colonics unit over her bathtub. Now she can give herself a colonic any time she wants.

She phoned me recently with a question. During her colonics, white fluid like milk was gushing out. She wanted to know if this was a bad sign.

"How does it smell afterwards?" I asked.

"Rotten ... putrid," she replied.

"How do you feel after the white stuff comes out?" I asked.

"Incredible," she answered, "Really wonderful."

The same white fluid had come out from my colon too after about 500 colonics on myself. I also felt wonderful afterwards. What is it? I would guess that it is some kind of liquid mucus trapped between the colon wall and the putrid lining of fecal matter which eventually wears thin, allowing the "milk" to flow out. We both experienced about half a gallon of it filling the tubing in a rush, like a damn had broken inside, with a sense of relief difficult to explain. Perhaps the closest experience to it I've had is holding my breath under water for a long time and then surfacing to take a big breath.

If colon hygiene released only brown fecal matter, that would be beneficial in its own right. However, after a person commits to their wellness and exerts the sustained effort required for deep internal cleansing, really bizarre stuff starts flowing out with the water. I don't know many people who have done as many colonics on themselves as I have. I stopped counting at 700 and probably have done another 500 since then.

Understand, my friend, I have taken myself through the process, which gives me a unique qualification. I have seen what leaves the body after 700 colonics and it looks nothing like what exits after one or two colonics.

After each colonic I asked myself:

"Do you feel better?"

"Do you look better?"

"Would you want what was removed back inside your body?"

My answers were always, yes, yes, no. So I kept going. I once drove an old motorcycle to Alaska using the same logic. If I could drive it around the block, why couldn't I drive a thousand miles?

When Dr. Jensen wrote his book about 25 years ago, one year probably was a good rule of thumb for healing the colon. Some estimate today that it requires 15 colonics for every year of your life on the planet. When I first started cleansing I never would have agreed to that figure and recall thinking I was "clean" after 45 colonics, then after 100 and about a dozen more times after that, times I felt significantly clean.

Not to discourage anybody, but after five years of bowel cleansing, at age 47, and converting to a diet of mostly raw fruits, vegetables, nuts, and seeds for several months, my bowel is finally snapping back into shape. Previously I had thought I was healthy, that I didn't have a constipation problem although I ate fast food almost daily, and I had never had a serious disease. So I was healthy, right?

"Some estimate today that it requires 15 colonics for every year of your life on the planet."

There is not one doubt in my mind that if I hadn't taken up bowel cleansing, I would be sick and dying today. For some reason I have been given a second opportunity to live. With that has come the awareness that America is still a wonderful land full of possibility and joy.

This is also why I found the doctor's reply on the Oprah show to be so insulting and insidious. That white milk inside an unhealthy colon eats baby aspirin for breakfast.

In summary: Colon cleansing will take you longer than you might expect, but you should feel better after each session along the way. What comes out of you might be surprising, especially if you believe you are healthy and don't need colonics. If you get to the level where white milk comes out, feel free to consult your doctor, although he or she will most likely have no idea what you are talking about. That's when you realize you have entered the forest at the darkest point and suddenly life is an adventure and you feel the wind in your hair and you have my permission at this point to scream "Yeehaw!" at the top of your lungs.

Are you buying in?

Consumers still hold the cards when it comes to the American system. Not voters, consumers. Writing your senator is secondary to what you buy. Two next door neighbors can have the same senator and totally opposite buying habits.

Buying into "the system" of typical American farming and food-making with your hard-earned dollars means you buy into chronic illness. It involves a conscious choice.

Media supports the corporate raid that saps your strength. For example, *Prevention* Magazine is a bizarre example of preventative health. Can the editors really be serious printing this short blurb?

How Twinkies conquer stress:
"Skip the guilt -- new research suggests we're hardwired to reach for sweet stuff when the going gets tough. Your agitated ancestors grabbed berries after the marauding tigers slunk away; you head for the candy machine after the boss roars. 'You need to refuel for the next crisis,' explains study co-author Norman Pecoraro, PhD." (p. 48, March '04)

That looks a lot more like *permission* than prevention -- if not downright promotion! How about these headlines in the same issue?

- **WHY REAL MEN NEED MILK**
  One in four guys over 50 will break a bone because of osteoporosis.

- **Low-sodium jerky at last!**

- **Relax: Cola won't break your bones**

- **Who says nothing good comes in a microwave tray?**

- **Kids Need Cholesterol Checks Too**
  Who needs a check? Kids age 2 or older ..."

Advertising in this same issue are pharmaceutical makers who -- just guessing -- may have investments in snack foods, dairy products, beef, cola, and drugs to lower cholesterol. These advertisers in one issue include Aventis, the American Dairy Farmers and Milk Processors, Allegra, Bristol-Myers Squibb, Prevacid, Aricept (for Alzheimer's) made by Pfizer, Pepcid AC made by Johnson and

Johnson, Purina, Synvisc (for osteoarthritis) made by Wyeth, Kraft Foods, Nexium, Botox, Humira (for arthritis), Jell-O, Kelloggs, Zelnorm, Singulair, "Once Daily" Arimidex (for breast cancer "prevention"), Ecotrin (aspirin) and last but not least of these major advertisers in *Prevention*, the state of Texas.

Anyway, let's just say *Prevention* Magazine has a few advertisers to please, many of whom have bought 2 to 3 page spreads to accommodate the list of drug side effects.

The question is -- Are you buying it?

More on the media's dumbing down

After I had learned more about health, I found it amazing how little there was of correct information being presented in the mainstream media. So I got on the phone and contacted a reporter at my town's daily newspaper, *The Tennessean*.

"I think I have made some discoveries about health," I told him.

"Are you a doctor?"

"I think I know why fiber is not helping people with constipation or preventing precancerous growths in clinical studies."

"No," I replied, "Just a common ordinary citizen who has stumbled onto some things that *Tennessean* readers should know."

"Like what?" he asked.

"Like I think I know why Americans get osteoporosis and how to prevent getting it," I replied.

"What else?" he asked.

"I think I know why fiber is not helping people with constipation or preventing precancerous growths in clinical studies," I said. "Did you read the article you published on fiber last year?"

"No," he said. "Is that all?"

"There's more -- what if your readers are taking pain medications for arthritis, yet those very pills are accelerating the arthritic condition?"

"And you think we should write an article on that," he said.

"Definitely!" I replied. "This is news ... about health. You report on health, right? Did you know that doctors are prescribing cholesterol-lowering drugs that deplete the muscle tissue of Coenzyme Q10, a vital heart nutrient? Are you aware of how deficiencies in CoQ10 contribute to heart disease?"

"No," he said, "Can you provide me with documentation?"

I got so excited I could barely contain myself. I rushed him a packet of information to get him started investigating these concerns. He phoned me back saying that he wanted to do a story on *me*, about colon hygiene. He visited my office and try as I might to engage him in conversation about health issues confronting my clients, he expressed no interest in my findings. In fact, he became quite critical, asking questions to put me on the defense of colon hygiene.

Finally I said, "Is this article intended to run me out of town?"

Suddenly he perked up. People's energy betrays them. Everything up until that point of our conversation had been totally low in energy.

The story ran in October of '03. The headline was: **Straight Flush Beats a Full Colon**, quite clever. The article's sub-headline read: *Interest in colon hydrotherapy picks up despite lack of proven medical benefits*. The cut line under my photo read, "Although there's no medical evidence of any benefits from rinsing out the colon, it's becoming increasingly popular." Stated within the article: "There's no medical evidence that colon hydrotherapy, also known as colonics, colon irrigation, or high colonics, provides any benefits."

I sent an email to the reporter suggesting that the only reason that there's "no proven medical benefits" is because there are no medical *studies* on colon hydrotherapy. I asked him what studies he was referring to and I asked him why no mention was made of the broader issues I had raised.

The reporter's response was that the article was an initial coverage of colon hydrotherapy and that the issues I had raised would be covered in future articles. Two years have passed. So much for local news reporting.

It's difficult for me to understand how the media became so dull. Take just about any subject of fantastic importance and the stories in mainstream media veer into the most irrelevant aspects within fifteen seconds and I'm thinking, "What benefit do I get exposing myself to these dumb ideas?"

I can't figure it out except to wonder if they write the stories so stupidly to make the advertising stand out more. Like compared to the article *The Tennessean* wrote on colon hygiene, women's shoes look smart.

Chapter Five
Ted, his Godzilla fistula, and other client tales

We've all heard the expression, "Only her hairdresser knows for sure." Likewise, a colon hygienist knows certain things, special things. Normal, healthy-looking people reveal secrets to me, mostly, that they are falling apart.

One client was the kind of person you would want for a next door neighbor. He listed his illnesses and prescriptions like reading a shopping list and finally shrugged saying he had a prostate problem with minor incontinence. The problem kept him awake at night. I wanted to throw him over my shoulder in a fireman's carry to somewhere. Where? Another time, another place.

A second client, Ted, has a disease of the gut stemming from diverticulitis. This illness is a pouch (or pouches) which protrudes from the colon wall appearing like a mushroom. It is chronically inflamed, like an angry internal pimple the size of your thumb. This type of inflamed pouch pressed against Ted's bladder and literally melted a hole in it creating a fistula. Then an opening formed between these two organs such that he experienced hard fecal matter (and gas) passing out his penis.

Ouch!

"According to a recent Cornell University study, 84 percent of consumers are either confused about healthy eating or have given up trying to make sense of it all."

Before Ted, I thought I had heard it all. He explained that this illness is more common than you would know because if you had it, you would vow secrecy while rushing to surgery.

The irony is that Ted is a bit of a health nut. He has been a vegetarian since 1970. According to a recent Cornell University study, 84 percent of consumers are either confused about healthy eating or have given up trying to make sense of it all. If you knew Ted, his condition was truly confusing. If a vegetarian diet resulted in a rotten gut, why even try? (Note: Ted consumed lots and lots of cheese.)

If you are a colon hygienist with half a brain, you realize that the clients who use your services represent a cross-section of society. For every guy who comes to see you with incontinence or poop passing out his penis, there are 99 just like him who are staying home and not getting colonics. For every female client with chronic bladder or yeast infections, there are 99 not getting colonics.

You have a face to go with the statistics. If I read that antidepressant sales are at an all-time high of $1 billion dollars per month in the U.S., I can picture my clients who take antidepressants with all their surrounding circumstances. Approaching five years as a colon hygienist and ten years as a massage therapist, I've heard most of the stories going around. I can enter a crowded restaurant and sit amidst a buzzing happy scene and perceive the underlying chaos and sorrow. Snap your fingers and I can become as happy as the rest and still not sacrifice professional awareness.

I tune to public radio one day and hear a story about skin cancer. The reporter states that fifty-percent of those with skin cancer get it a second time and of those, 75-percent will get it a third time. If I could phone in and explain why this happens, I would. But I know they wouldn't take my call because I have already read about the close connection between skin cancer and a toxic colon in a book available to anybody. But to the radio reporter, these statistics are shrouded in mystery.

I know now that you could pick any random person off the street, give them two colonic sessions, and remove ten feet of fecal matter. Vegetarians have poop that is slightly softer than meat-eaters, but the volume is still there. And a large gut is not a sign of lots of poop. Skinny people are just as backed-up.

Let's do this: bring me any random person off the street. Have them stop eating solid food for two days, the amount of time doctors say it takes to pass any and all stool. I will then remove ten feet of fecal matter from their gut in two colonic sessions. And if we only get out five feet, that still is *five* feet.

You are any random person. That volume of poop is in you. It goes with you to bed and arises with you in the morning. You don't poop anything near five feet long, do you? Brush your teeth and change your underwear and then it leaves the house with you.

What is it doing there? Is it normal and natural? Does it make you feel heavy and sluggish? Could it cause internal pouches of inflammation in your gut?

Only your colon hygienist knows for sure.

Rachel needs enlightenment

The first step toward wellness is to picture yourself well. The second step is then to do whatever you want.

You can't *try* to be well. Effort spoils the equation.

The first time I met my client, Rachel, she sat down and asked me, "I eat half a birthday cake every day. Do you think that is okay?"

This woman was smooth! What a trap she set before me. I responded by saying, "Yes, of course! I think you should eat all the birthday cake you want."

"You do?" she asked, "I've never heard that before."

"Well, Rachel, have you ever followed anybody's advice?"

"No," she replied, "I guess not."

"Then eat all the cake you want," I said.

Thing was, Rachel really did want me to give her advice. She needed something to buck up *against*. I refused to play that role.

She would come in and say, "I ate half a birthday cake last night."

"Good," I replied.

Or once she said, "I ate six honey bunnies yesterday."

"Good!"

Some people must be told what to do so they can then do what they want. Let's not play games. Let's skip directly to your doing what you want.

Another client was talking with me during her colonic and the topic turned to the magnetic power of thoughts. I said, "Human emotions possess higher magnetism than thoughts," and my client replied, "Exactly!" I said, "There are scientific measurement devices that register emotions on a scale, positive being strong and negative being weak," and my client replied: "I know that!"

"Really?" I exclaimed, "Do you know which emotion records the highest?"

"Enlightenment," she said smiling because she knew the answer.

"I wonder what registers second highest," I said, not expecting an answer.

"Joy," she replied.

"Yes, that does make sense," I said, "Do you know what vibrates the lowest?"

She paused two seconds and replied: "Shame."

If you think about the steps toward health, picturing yourself well should give you butterflies and joy, which has a strong magnetic attraction and puts you in the realm of seeing miracles. "Doing what you want" means eating all the birthday cake you want, all the fast food double-meat hamburgers you want, smoking all the cigarettes you want, drinking all the beer you want, or taking all the drugs you want, legal or otherwise. If shame provides a low magnetic power, you will not attract health through shame.

Bless all of your choices. Understanding this is a form of enlightenment. I'll say it again: Bless all of your choices. That is enlightenment at its best. Anybody can bless things. And then comes joy.

The thought of such simplicity could have you smiling.

Are you better every day?

One of my favorite clients has been Pam. When I met her several years ago, her eye sockets were hollow like pictures you see of people from a Nazi concentration camp. She weighed 85 pounds. She pooped an average of once per week.

Though she was only age 46, Pam lived in a nursing home. Part of our arrangement was that I would give her a ride to and from my office, not far. She came twice a week. Initially we spent our time together in silence.

After a month, Pam began to open up. Mostly she ranted and raved about her illness. I would keep quiet and listen. One day I could take no more. I said to her, "Pam, I believe that two people have the ability to support each other in bringing good things into their lives. Or they can support each other that things are bad. If I listen to you talk about how sick you are and I don't respond, then that means that I am supporting you being ill. Is that what you want?"

"No," she replied.

"Then it's wrong for us to concentrate on your illness," I explained.

She retracted back into silence, which I wouldn't allow her to do either. I said, "Pam, I want you to say: 'I am getting better every day.'"

She just stared at me.

"I mean, Pam, I want you to say it right *now*," I said.

She bucked up and replied, "I don't know that I *am* getting better --"

I had built enough trust with her to interrupt her saying, "*Say it!*"

Almost inaudibly she said, "I'm getting better."

"Better EVERY DAY," I entreated her.

"I'm getting better every day," she said barely above a whisper.

Later that same day my phone rang. It was Pam. It didn't sound like her and it took me a second to understand what she was shouting -- "Scott Webb I AM GETTING BETTER EVERY DAY!!"

"What?" I said.

"You told me to say that I am getting better every day and I am," Pam said, "I feel better ... I am better ... I know that it's true!"

Honestly, that moment was a crowning achievement for me and it can still make me shed a tear of joy to think about it.

One of the services I perform with most colonic sessions is a quick foot rub. The first session with Pam revealed sores on her calves and feet, like pink Dalmatian spots, like plastic patches you could peel off, very bizarre. Pam explained that she had had them for several years and nothing the doctors gave her had helped.

After a month of colonics, however, they started disappearing. Soon they were totally gone without fanfare.

Another improvement with Pam -- she began gaining weight. At a hundred pounds she complained she was fat, which of course she wasn't. Eventually Pam went to 115 pounds and became well enough that she moved out of the nursing home into an apartment complex next to my office so she could walk to her appointments. After a year of living there she finally moved back home to live with her father on their family farm in Clarksville, Tennessee.

Noteworthy about Pam's transition toward wellness is that her initial condition was too severe for an ordinary colonic. Most colon therapists provide sessions lasting fifteen to twenty minutes long. Pam's sessions required at *minimum* one hour. It's back breaking and boring work, like fishing while leaning over the boat waiting for a bite.

The first time she came, I believe that it had been three weeks since Pam had a bowel movement. The first forty minutes of her session, nothing came out. But her gut ballooned out like she had swallowed a basketball. At this point, I had no clue what to do. If you've ever been rock climbing, you know the feeling -- can't go up, can't go down, not either way side-ways, so you stop to think. That's what I did with Pam.

"I believe that it had been three weeks since Pam had a bowel movement. The first forty minutes of her session, nothing came out."

Suddenly, she exploded. My tubing shuddered as foul wave after wave gushed forth, even spilling around the scope, ruining the towel. It was unbelievable. What I noticed, as the volcano quieted, was Pam's face. It glowed with a smile and she said, "I feel better."

I purchased some cotton pads from a discount store and Pam's initial sessions soiled half a dozen pads, like bailing water from a sinking ship. Each time I was rewarded when Pam would say, "Thank you, Scott." One time the tubing filled four times end to end, which equates to roughly fifteen feet of poop, from a woman weighing under a hundred pounds. Astounding! Normally I don't smell anything, but with Pam, let's just say the odor served to further motivate me -- to remove the source of it.

People have told me that colonics can harm your health. I say, *Bah!*

I personally believe, and think Pam's family would agree, Pam was deathly ill when she first came for colonics. If she had seen another colon hygienist, if they would have seen her as a client at all, and had Pam gotten the standard twenty-minute colonic, she may have not improved and may have died. But her condition was already extremely advanced and the many doctors she had seen were not helping her with or without colonics. Pam's experience alone had me convinced -- colonics are good. Or at least I have not once had a client respond, "That was bad for me."

The other dumb thing I hear is that a person will become dependent on colonics. Not just with Pam, but with every client, cleaning the colon makes it work <u>better</u>.

A female client age 45 just came to me saying her doctor told her she had a "lazy colon." I couldn't help but laugh. "Was that his diagnosis?" I asked her.

"Yes, a *lazy* colon."

As a colon therapist, I am not allowed to discuss with my clients their doctor's diagnosis. But what we are looking at here, as a point in a book, is not a lazy colon, but an overworked colon. A colon chronically carrying fifteen feet of fecal matter, as in Pam's case, simply gives up. That does not make the colon lazy. Just a realist.

Fact is, Pam's colon became awakened after increasing to three colonic sessions per week for one year. Her leaking stopped. She began using the toilet on days between sessions. She never could have moved home if her colon hadn't been cleaned and working again, stronger and better than ever.

One final point on Pam. You may not know this, but doctors are the only profession in America allowed to diagnose disease. This ability is rigidly protected by the American Medical Association and as far as I am concerned, they can have it.

First, "to diagnose" means that somebody is the expert and somebody else is the dumb recipient. It not only broadly assumes that any diagnosis is correct, it assumes that all those with a medical degree are equally capable of performing the diagnostic process.

What the medical profession has done is the same thing that the fast food industry has done: Limit every possibility for error. How the fast food industry has done this is to create a mechanized robot-type work where people perform the most simple tasks of input and output. Doctors and hospitals and insurance companies have done the same thing. It's moved medicine into the field of button-pushing and computer print-outs. It's less for the benefit of the patient, more for the protection of the industry, because the insurance business is well aware that all doctors, as those who diagnose, are not created equally. Therefore, uniformity has become the tool of the new medicine and guess what? Nothing is more uniform than a print-out and a pill.

Second, this has created a huge gaping hole where people complaining of illness turn up with no illness. One client came to me after not having a bowel movement for 19 days. She previously had gone to the emergency room. Doctors there ran a battery of tests costing $5,000 and they came in the room with good news -- they had found nothing wrong. She said, "But I haven't gone to the bathroom in 19 days! Can you at least give me an enema?" To which the nurse replied, "I am not giving you an enema!"

If the medical paradigm (of uniform illness, uniform tests) becomes out-of-sync with changes in culture, then many, many illnesses will not show up in the lab. When the patient insists they are ill, then a surgery is often performed, often with no improvement. You can have your gall bladder removed by a robot, but that won't mean you're well.

Now there are exceptions all the way around. One exceptional case does not make a trend. What's happening is that exceptions to previous trends are now large enough to form their own group and many of these people become my clients.

Third, one diagnosis these days generally leads to a second illness. There is a *pattern* to diagnosis that medicine refuses to track and observe. Even *I* can see this. These patterns are evolving into social issues, something for a sociologist to report, and they will, because the group of uninsured in America has grown so large that states and the federal government are taking up the slack, even municipal governments, and they are now observing the social costs of bad diagnosis and a spiraling of disease.

"Doctors are the only profession in America allowed to diagnose disease."

Lastly, the worst thing about "diagnosis" is that it forges an agreement between the patient and the doctor. It takes two for this tango. As long as everybody agrees that somebody is ill, it's that much tougher for the power of healing to occur. For a while, the Christian preachers were onto the power of agreement, but you don't hear much about it any more. Perhaps creating a better way for medical people to relate with patients will be medicine's next frontier. In other words, robotics has reached diminishing returns.

Do you want to be well? It's quite simple. Say, "*I am getting better every day! Everything I do and everyone around me helps me to be well.*" Acting the skeptic has never improved the odds. You must want health, envision it, demand it, and shout it for everybody to hear.

Even be the fool for it. Shout it right now: "I am getting better EVERY DAY!"

Nurse Mo questions vaccines

My client Maureen came to see me. She asked me, "What's new?"

"I've just finished reading a book by Kevin Trudeau," I replied. "Have you heard of him?"

"No, what does he write about?"

"Mostly about the failings of medicine," I explained, "He says, 'It's all about the money.'"

"*What's* all about the money?" she asked.

"Medicine."

Mo laughed, "It *is* all about the money."

About now I notice that she's come from work and is wearing scrubs and I remember that Mo is a nurse. When you've known somebody a long time you tend to forget their profession. She shares her experience working at a children's hospital as the front nurse.

"When I first started nursing, I was shocked by the number of children brought to the emergency room with seizures, Grand mal seizures," she begins. The common element she found was that often the children had been recently vaccinated. She read the medical literature on her own and discovered that one of the side effects of vaccinations was Grand mal seizures. For her, this was a detail missed by the hospital doctors and she brought this to the attention of one of the doctors. The doctor said, "Vaccines are *not* causing seizures."

When she persisted, she was told not to discuss it any more. I asked her, "You mean you were brought into an office and told not to talk about it?"

"Yes, that is exactly what I mean."

"And you shut up?"

"You bet!"

"Why?"

"Because I wanted to keep my job."

"How many kids were having seizures?" I ask.

"Over the course of years I worked there -- hundreds," she replies.

"How can that be happening?"

She explains that seizures are underreported because doctors are not collecting data based as a side-effect of vaccines, but as general seizures. Not only is it difficult to prove in court that a vaccine might have caused the seizure, but she says that the U.S. government has made it so the pharmaceutical companies making the vaccines are not liable. Back a generation ago, the liability was so high for those making vaccines that they threatened not to make them. The government took on the liability and added a tax to the cost of vaccines to pay families who had a child suffer or die from an adverse reaction.

"So the government did the right thing," I comment.

"No," she says, "It's all about the money."

"Huh?" I reply, to which she makes a face telling me to figure it out for myself.

"I see," I say slowly, "The government has created an umbrella of protection ..." Mo nods for me to continue. "And the pharmaceutical industry receives income for every child born, like a tax in the form of a vaccine ... so if you multiplied every child born -- times thirty dollars -- that comes to a huge sum in pharmaceutical bills."

"Thirty dollars?" Mo exclaims, "You haven't priced vaccines recently. We're talking *hundreds* of dollars before the baby even gets home from the hospital. First thing a baby experiences right out of the womb is a Hepititus B vaccine and children don't even get Hepititus B." She then rattles off the seven vaccinations a child receives by the age of two months and then seven more at four months and then ...

I interrupt her, "I don't think my kids had that many vaccinations."

"Exactly," she says, "They didn't. The number keeps going up, up and up. You should investigate it. There are lots of great books written on it."

"First thing a baby experiences right out of the womb is a Hepititus B vaccine and children don't even get Hepititus B."

"I'm not really writing about vaccines," I explain, "Except if it illustrates the general madness."

"Trust me," she says, "It's madness. The new doctor interns don't think for themselves. They *can't* think for themselves. It drives me crazy."

"But we're talking about intelligent people," I interject.

"It's all about the money," she must point out again. "Did you know that most doctors won't see a child who's parents refuse vaccines? Schools enforce it too. The pharmaceutical industry has an iron grip on the situation. They are the most profitable of all manufacturers and the most protected by the U.S. government."

"Is this one big drug company?" I ask.

"No, the field is highly competitive. There's lots of *big* money in drugs and vaccines."

"And the government pays families if their child has an adverse reaction?" I ask.

"Are you kidding?" Mo laughs, "You have to PROVE to the government that the vaccine caused a bad reaction. They make it so tough most people can't handle the process. Doctors are legally bound to report adverse reactions like Grand mal seizures, but there's no penalty if they don't. You would be hard-pressed to find a doctor who would go against the pharmaceutical industry. And whatever numbers are reported to the government are kept tight under lock and key," she says.

Anyway, people talk to me during their colonic session. We just talk. I don't have any agenda except that I feel curious about people. About a dozen nurses come to see me for colon therapy and I sometimes pick their brains.

That's all on that. Unless of course Americans get mandated to get vaccinated against something like bird flu. Just think of the bucks for those clucks!

David's medical records

David showed up at my office for a colonic session carrying a three-inch thick folder holding copies of his medical records. He offered to have me review his file in case it would be helpful to his receiving colonics.

"No," I said, "That's not necessary. Colon hygiene is not a medical treatment and what I'm doing has nothing to do with your medical history."

During his session, he shared his story with me. He's from a small town outside Nashville where he has been active in his community, particularly as a beloved baseball coach. He coached his doctor's son and had a friendly relationship with his doctor for many years.

After David's father became seriously ill last year, he decided to avoid a similar fate and lose some major weight at age 47. He started at 278 pounds and proceeded to drop ninety pounds within one year.

David opened his folder and showed me test results from October, 2004. His total cholesterol was 183; LDL was 117 and triglycerides, 173. Checked was to "Continue Current Treatment and Medications." The doctor's comment was, *"Your diabetes is really bad! If you do not make the necessary changes, you will require insulin."*

What happened next is that David came across a book by Robert Young, "The pH Miracle." From this reading, David changed to a more alkaline diet of increased raw fruits and vegetables. On January 18, 2005, he saw his doctor again.

His test results included a drop in total cholesterol to 129; LDL to 73 and triglycerides, 91. At the bottom of the report is two words: *"Much improved."*

David's doctor told him at this time that he was happy to see that the current treatment and medications were working so well. He replied, "No, Doc, I quit taking that stuff back in October." He explained that his improvements came from natural means.

His doctor cautioned him that natural supplements included heavy amounts of mercury and would damage his health. David saw through this lie and replied, "The real poisons are right there in that closet that holds your samples of medicines you hand out."

The doctor then made a few notes and left the room. David then received a **certified** letter from his doctor (and family friend) dated February 10, 2005. It reads:

Re: Primary Care
Mr. Mayberry,

After reviewing your records I feel it would be in your best medical interest to keep with one primary care provider. With this in mind and your belief in holistic medicine you should transfer all your medical care to this individual.

I will continue to be your primary care physician for 30-days from this date and you will need to transfer all your medical records to this caregiver.

Sincerely,
C.T., M.D.

David now picked my brain on colonics with unrestrained ferocity. I recommended that he read Dr. Bernard Jensen's books on colon health. David decided to receive five colonic sessions and showed up for his second session with one of Dr. Jensen's books already half-read. Dr. Jensen is "old school." His information was decades-old, but still relevant. He advocated using a colema board for internal cleansing which today is not widely used because colonics have become more the mainstay.

One of my clients had given me a colema board which was sitting at home in a closet. I offered it to David for free and he was anxious to have it. Next I knew he was using it for additional internal cleansing at home.

One benefit of colon hygiene is that it improves dark circles under the eyes. David has these circles along with puffiness and a purple tint. This translates as liver toxicity, colon impaction, a congested lymphatic system, and internal inflammation. By cleansing the colon, the lymphatic system and liver can dump its waste for removal and assist the body in healing internal inflammation. Bottom line: better appearance.

I haven't had the luxury of reviewing a client's files other than getting a general impression of their health by looking at their face, skin tone, listening to their conversation, and of course, noting the way their poop exits, its texture and the color of the water that flows out with it. Just as Eskimos have many words for "snow," a colonic therapist easily could have a dozen words for "poop."

On 12/06/04, David underwent an MRI for his liver and abdomen. What they found was noted on a report: "There is a 2.5 cm mildly peripherally enhancing poorly defined mass in the right liver lobe. 2 probable small cysts within the spleen. Small simple cysts in both kidneys."

Noted on a test result dated 12/15/04 was a description of his colonoscopy procedure. It reads, "The split-flexible colonscope was then inserted and retroflexed. Internal hemorrhoids were noted. The scope was advanced ... This area was 'riddled' with diverticular changes as was the descending and transverse colon."

Just as Eskimos have many words for "snow," a colonic therapist easily could have a dozen words for "poop."

David also had another operation on 12/15, an EGD. During this they found "mild distal esophagitis" and small ulcerations of the gastric cardia.

On a pathology report dated 12/21/04, the comment reads: "The primary finding in this liver is the presence of a chronic portal hepatitis with increased connective tissue in the portal tracts."

What does all this jargon mean? Basically, as of December, 2004, David was falling apart. His internal organs had abnormal growths and ulcers and his colon was "riddled" with pockets of inflammation and internal hemorrhoids. It's a "before" snapshot of his insides that were producing chronic abdominal pain and exhaustion.

The "after" picture remains to be taken. So far we see that David's doctor wants no part of the process if it means David might actually become healthy. We're talking -- healthy from the inside-out. David looks better on the outside, which reflects the state of his insides. And he did it all on his own. Dude deserves a *high five*.

His process toward wellness has not been perfect, but then whose is?

One other note: natural herbs and supplements do <u>not</u> contain high amounts of mercury. If your doctor makes this claim, insist on receiving a written list of specific supplements he or she believes contain mercury and the exact clinical studies which support this. If the doctor balks, find a new doctor. If the doctor stalls, request this information within one week and have it put into writing that it has been stated that natural health supplements contain "dangerous metals" to be substantiated with proof.

For a doctor to use his or her position to make wild statements not supported by clinical studies borders on malpractice. Hold their feet to the fire, same as they are holding patient's feet to the fire when they pursue natural means for health.

What does contain toxic doses of mercury? For decades, vaccines have contained mercury as a preservative. Some hemorrhoidal suppositories contain mercury. Metal fillings in teeth contain mercury. Fish caught in polluted ocean waters contain mercury, particularly large predatory fish like shark and tuna.

What does mercury do inside the human body? It ain't pretty. It facilitates yeast overgrowth in the gut and internal inflammation. The only natural supplement I am aware which might contain mercury would be fish oil supplements and most likely, not. Otherwise, our water supply and our medicines potentially could have mercury in it and natural supplements would not.

For more specific information, ask your doctor.

Roy recommends a doctor's advice

Roy is *not* the sort of person you would imagine receiving regular colonic treatments. He is a white male nearing retirement with a net worth in the millions of dollars. He started his industrial services company from the ground up, the kind of hard-nosed, no-nonsense guy who drives a big fancy car and plays golf and tennis.

Knowing that I am writing a book on colon hygiene, Roy tells me that I must write it *with* a doctor to receive the necessary credibility. He tells me that his doctor has stated that beyond 48 hours, nothing gets permanently stuck inside the colon.

Roy has heard the process of how I formulated this book. Initially I wrote an article comparing digestion to composting and I submitted it to organic farming publications explaining how corporate farming using massive amounts of chemicals has constipated Americans. One of America's foremost eco-farming newsletters, *Acres USA*, found it intriguing and published it in their April, 2004 issue. The cover story of that issue is titled, *'Sound Science' Is Killing Us*. My kind of publication.

From my published article I received the attentions of four

literary agents. One stated that I would need a writing partner with established credentials to capture the interest of a major book publisher. She asked for permission to forward my article to one of her authors who had written a book about digestive disorders for Harvard Medical School. Then I received an email from her author stating his interest to collaborate on the project.

"Yes, but is he a *doctor*?" Roy asked me.

"No," I replied.

"You must write this with a doctor," Roy insists, "It's the only way people will believe you."

I explain to him that Bernard Jensen, the "father of colon hygiene," was a doctor and he has already written decades ago about the many health benefits of internal cleansing. And a recent book is written by a former colon hygienist in collaboration with a doctor titled: *Gut Solutions -- Natural Solutions to Your Digestive Problems.*

"That's what you need too," Roy says emphatically, "A doctor backing you."

"My work is sociology, not pharmacology."

I explain to him that doctors are required to work by a formula that no longer works and that my book introduces a new formula that says most people can be totally well without medications. It shifts the focus of wellness from relying on disinterested "experts" to individual self-empowerment and creative thinking. "The very nature of medicine thwarts empowerment," I tell him. "My work is sociology, not pharmacology."

During a recent session I announce to Roy that I will most likely self-publish my material.

"I'd like to help you financially," he says.

"But I am not writing this with a doctor," I state.

"I know," he shrugs.

"Then why would you want to help me?" I ask.

Almost apologetically he replies: "Because I understand everything you have told me and I believe you are right."

When to eat French fries

I had a client who lives near me call and ask me to take her to the emergency room at the hospital. She was feeling nauseous and sweating following a surgery and somewhat in a panic. When I got there she was in tears. I drove her to the hospital, but left after another friend came to sit with her until they looked her over and sent her home.

In the morning she called with another favor. She was still feeling ill, but had a craving for French fries. She asked if I would bring her some fries.

"No," I said, "What if one of my clients were to see me at McDonald's?"

"Oh, I see what you mean," she replied.

"I'm just kidding," I said.

I ordered her the larger size because I thought I might want to steal a few fries. But then to my surprise they smelled bad to me so I didn't eat any.

When I got to her place, she offered me a cigarette. Now I hadn't smoked a cigarette for some time and this sounded good to me, so I accepted. She ate her fries sitting on her bed while I smoked a cigarette.

The thing is -- you can be too healthy for your own good. We all have unhealthy cravings and it's not always bad to yield. I think it's far worse to get judgmental and imagine yourself too pure for this old world.

How some people die

"It was Einstein who first stirred up the scientific world when he claimed that substance and matter are convertible. He declared that the formed and unformed worlds are made out of the same energy. Start realizing that nothing can stand between you and that good that you dare to choose mentally and radiate outward through your thoughts, feelings, words and expectancies."

Catherine Ponder

Bob came to me a very sick man. His face was ash gray. One look at him and you could tell something was seriously wrong. He was in his late fifties. Each breath came with much effort.

During his colonics, he told me stories from his life, some funny, others tragic. He told me of his love for the swamp country of South Carolina, where the copperhead snakes lay in the afternoon sun shimmering.

Bob was so backed-up that nothing came out during his first session except gas. And I mean *lots* of gas, at least a gallon of it. It blew the tubing dry, which is unusual. He felt so much better that he paid for three sessions.

Bob ended up coming for six sessions before I told him he could get colonics at no charge. He needed to come more frequently, but had become so weak he couldn't drive and his wife worked at a day care center and money was tight. He also had no health insurance and the doctors told him there was nothing wrong with him, but I suspect he had an advanced case of cancer and there was little to be done for him.

At times Bob expressed incredible anger and many resentments. I once asked him what he had to live for. It took him a long time to reply. "I'm not sure," he said.

"If you did have something to live for, what would that be," I asked.

"I'd like to have a farm some day," he replied, "With chickens."

"Chickens?" I asked, "Tell me about your chickens."

"Oh, I don't know," he said vacantly.

"Bob," I said seriously, "You have got to really want those chickens. I believe your life depends on it at this point."

"It was just a thought," he said.

"I once asked him what he had to live for. It took him a long time to reply."

I received a call that weekend from Bob's wife. She was at the hospital and asked if I could come down to sit with her. Bob was dead. He had fallen asleep on the couch and died in his sleep. "He has no friends," she said, "And you were a friend to him."

I drove to sit with her at the hospital. I held her hand while she wept. Bob illustrated how life can wear a person down and then momentum carries them over the edge. In other words, energy and matter are convertible.

Does anger convert into matter?

I had another client, Rick, in his early fifties with advanced liver cancer. He told me that he had everything to live for and was going to beat his cancer. Rick was tough like an old Marine drill sergeant. But little by little, Rick wore down just like Bob.

Rick found that colonics helped him feel better, but nearing the end he was going down fast. His doctor had given him less than a month to live. Rick held out for about four. I installed a colonics unit in his home, but he was too weak to use it except once. I went to see him regardless, just in case he felt strong enough for a colonic. Rick differed from Bob in that he had lots of friends, family, and support.

What the two men did share was anger. Sometimes Rick would lash out at his private nurse in front of me, but they would both glance over in my direction and he would stop in mid sentence. A confidant told me that one of his frustrations came from people talking about his condition while they thought he was sleeping, saying stuff like, "He looks *ter*rible. I doubt he'll pull through the week," and "He's just not the same old happy-go-lucky guy."

One evening I received a phone call from Rick's business partner asking if I was available to sit with him in the hospital over night because his private nurse had called in sick. I agreed to it.

All night long Rick was restless and his mood violent. I walked him to the bathroom a couple of times and if he had been slightly stronger I have no doubt he would have punched me out for no reason whatsoever.

About 4 am I woke in my chair and saw him staring at me from his bed. He tried to say something, but his words were not intelligible. I put my ear close to his mouth and heard him ask me in a breathless whisper, "How ... could ... this ... happen?"

I wasn't positive he was serious, but his eyes begged me for a reply. I lied. "This happens to everybody," I said.

It doesn't need to happen. That is the truth. Cancer doesn't have to happen. But once you get cancer bad, at some point you can forget it. It's too late to make sense of it. So I expend my energy helping people to prevent it.

If I thought it would help anybody, I'd get angry too.

Chapter Six
Social Commentary on Katrina, New Orleans, etc.

The tragedy of New Orleans symbolizes the broad failure of the American system to protect its people. In the aftermath, Paul Krugman, a columnist for *The New York Times*, pointed out that <u>every</u> governmental safety agency has become woefully inadequate and underfunded. This includes the EPA (Environmental Protection Agency) and the FDA (Food and Drug Administration), not just the emergency agency, FEMA.

If you happened to catch the news five days after Hurricane Katrina hit the Gulf coast, then you witnessed for yourself residents still trapped in downtown New Orleans shouting for help. If the TV cameras filmed the clients who come to my office, you would witness a similar cry for help. Sick people are equally being failed today.

It's not that the American government has suddenly become thrift conscious. Take the subject of global warming. Whether you believe it to be a threat matters not. Just consider that if the mass usage of petroleum products can be shown to accelerate warming, then those who earn their living from petroleum products would oppose the very idea of "global warming." This relationship is an undisputed one-to-one.

"It's not that the American government has suddenly become thrift conscious."

It's easy to deny anything when government agencies created to protect humanity from such things have been gutted. Or programs are given progressive names like "Clean Air Act" while they serve an opposite function, giving corporations more leeway to pollute. Careful -- if you investigate this type of thing, it could horrify you.

We can observe that the oceans are indeed warming and ice is melting across the cold regions of the planet. And we know that the U.S. government has pulled out from the Kyoto Agreement, meaning that our government supports the burning of petroleum products. Now we are looking at vested interests and lots of dollars forming positions.

The same holds true with the FDA. We are looking at drug approval and safety monitoring based upon vested interests and lots of money. People die from adverse reactions to pharmaceutical drugs, the rough equivalent to a Katrina storm each and *every week*. The difference is that they die here and there, never in mass for the television cameras. The Vioxx scandal brought some of this to light, very briefly.

The last time pharmaceutical deaths were made public was in 1994, reported to be 106,000 annually in the U.S. These people basically took a medicine and keeled over. My sense is that it stopped being reported because it's gotten worse, not better.

We see vested interests also within the EPA. Lots of dollars can put pressure on the government's environmental position because dollars pay to put certain people into office so that safety comes second, profits first. Right now there is a rebellion within the EPA ranks over the safety of fluoride added to water supplies in America for over fifty years. It's proving to be a poison, with no benefit for teeth. It's akin to a hurricane's damage after you begin to see the ruined lives from drinking poison for decades.

What this means to you is that your government cannot be trusted to watch your back. That means you will need to rely on your friends and neighbors to get things done. Start talking with loved ones about these nationwide dangers to health.

This really isn't anything new. If it requires a hurricane to recognize it, that's sad, but better than nothing. If it takes you becoming chronically ill to prove it, that's not good either. If you feel terribly stuck, don't wait around. Get yourself unstuck.

Has health care become like *Saturday Night Live?*

I sat down to unwind in front of the TV and thought I was watching a rerun of *Saturday Night Live*. There were three cast members sitting in a news-like format taking calls from the public. The lady on the phone sounded totally victimized and whiny, like a Gilda Radner character in a comedy sketch.

But then I realized this was a real program.

The woman on the phone complained that her feet hurt at night and became so sensitive that nothing could touch them, not even the bed sheets. It kept her awake at night in fits of pain.

On the left sat a news moderator. To the right sat two doctors who looked so bored and disinterested by this woman's plight, it seemed unreal. One stared into space while the other played with his pen. The moderator was trying not to laugh. I mean she was biting-her-lip trying not to laugh and squirming in her seat.

If you had just flipped to the channel and thought it was *Saturday Night Live*, it might strike you as hilarious. The caller said her feet went numb and she couldn't find the gas pedal while driving, but she could find the brake. I know it's not funny, but watching the moderator fighting herself from busting out laughing, made me bust out.

The response of the doctors was also comical. Their replies demonstrated that they understood the caller's problem, in fact, commanded an impressive knowledge of her particular disease, the knowns and the unknowns, drugs for treatment, etc. Except -- *except* -- they offered her not a single shred of useful information.

Like if you changed the context and put those doctors in the caller's bedroom and she's complaining of severe foot pain, their textbook answers provided no relief whatsoever. Like if you had a bloody nose and two doctors sat in your room telling you about the various causes and possible treatments for blood coming out your nose, you would want to holler: *"Get me a cold, wet wash cloth, would you?!"*

Then a second caller came on. She had experienced similar excruciating foot pain, but had discovered that a pharmaceutical drug she had been taking to lower her cholesterol, a statin drug, CAUSED this pain. She explained that after she stopped taking the drug for

30 days, her foot sensitivity and numbness dissipated dramatically. The doctor then agreed with her, that certain drug reactions could trigger this type of painful reaction and that patients should review their medications and side effects with their doctor.

"After she stopped taking the drug for 30 days, her foot sensitivity and numbness dissipated dramatically."

Just before I flipped the channel, I heard the moderator say they had time for one more caller. At that point I really did want to watch an old rerun of *Saturday Night Live* because this health program was no longer funny.

The unhesitating public media

I was listening to Public Radio when I heard a story about new vaccines. Gosh -- it sounded horrible, a disease called meningitis. The vaccine was pitched as something every college freshmen should get and the commentator pointed out that supplies of it had been exhausted because of the demand, like some kind of national crisis. The story was flying at me so fast that I could barely catch the details except for -- "horrible disease" and "exhausted supplies" and "get it while you can."

The thing is, I've learned to take notes. So I reviewed what I had just heard. Meningitis is a RARE disease they said. In the United States, there are about 125 cases per year. Of that, 15 percent are fatal.

Well, do the math. What's 125 multiplied by 15 percent? Under 20 fatal cases per year out of how many *millions* they are saying should get the vaccine? But I hesitate to mention this because now MORE people will be wanting to get the meningitis vaccine. People hear "fatal" and rush to get vaccinated.

Observe your behavioral patterns when you hear about a disease and immediately want the vaccine against it. You would be more likely to win the lottery than catch meningitis. And you would be *way* more likely to die from a lightening bolt than from meningitis.

If someone could make a vaccine to protect against lightning strikes, everyone would want it. Even if one of the side-effects was that it made your feet hurt with excruciating pain at night. People will do crazy things. Including get a shot to prevent a disease they would never get in a million years.

And the media makes the whole thing quite sensational. The other half of the radio story was about whooping cough. They have a new vaccine for that also. It's called a "TDAP" shot in case you want that one too. I'm not sure, but it's probably in short supply, so you had better hurry.

Frosted children's health

I went on vacation this summer and spent a week living in the same house with my brother, his wife, their three kids aged between 8 and 13, and my sister and her five kids, also aged between 8 and 13, and my kids, ages 17 and 19.

My sister-in-law said first thing: "I'm glad we'll be living together because you can teach us how to eat healthy."

I love her dearly, but was forced to clarify: "You don't need *me* to tell you what's healthy and what's not."

During that week they ate their food and I ate mine with my kids. Of course there was some overlap. And I made every effort to love and not be the teacher, to share when appropriate, to withhold judgment, and to simply observe. I mean, I had forgotten what typical American kids eat.

For breakfast they ate frosted *Lucky Charms*. For lunch they ate leftover cake from the night before. For dinner they ate hot dogs.

After about three days of seeing this I took my sister aside. Her husband had died of cancer a year ago and the responsibility of raising five kids has been overwhelming. I said that she must find some way of getting real food into her kids or they would not fare well in the future, even the near future. Then I shut up and went into action.

I juiced organic carrots and kale and told each of her kids I would pay them one dollar per glass they would drink. Somehow these kids were getting nutrition!

"For breakfast they ate frosted *Lucky Charms*. For lunch they ate leftover cake from the night before. For dinner they ate hot dogs."

One of my nieces politely said, "Uncle Scott, I won't drink that for a dollar."

Rather than argue I asked, *"How much money do you want?"*

"FIVE dollars," she said thinking she would be exempt from drinking the juice.

"Okay," I said, "Five dollars then."

I watched her drink the juice and then I gave her five dollars. You know what? Kids are worth five dollars.

What are mental models?

When I worked as a magazine marketing manager, my supervisor often told me that the greatest leverage for industry improvement lay in the "mental models" of those running the organization. This language was foreign to me and I barely understood him until I got into the field of health. Then I realized that the greatest leverage a person has to improve their health depends on their mental models of health.

For example, if you get a cough and immediately think of taking cough medicine, that shows your mental model on treating a cough. Meanwhile, there might be another fifty reasonable options to treating and preventing a cough.

Another example: if a person's mental model of the human digestive system is that it eliminates all fecal matter in a timely manner, then the concept that the human body deteriorates from rotten poop within would never be accepted. From this belief other conclusions might be drawn based on that one assumption.

If poop actually does stick within, that turns all the tables.

Or consider my client who asked their doctor about the safety of colonics. If their mental model is that doctors know all, then whatever the doctor says will be believed. In this case the doctor said never to have a colonic because it could kill you.

Now if you were a colon hygienist, you would have a very different mental model about colonics.

"Mental models" might be confusing enough that you would rather not have any mental models (rather than have a wrong mental model), except that you have mental models about everything important to you. It's quite impossible to live in a neutral mental state and as you are reading this, my aim is to help equip you to examine your own assumptions about health.

"If poop actually does stick within, that turns all the tables."

And just as importantly, you must be able to recognize the mental models of others who would seek to give you their opinions.

For example, if somebody told you that there are four million rats living on the island of Manhattan, you should ask, "How were they counted?" Otherwise you will believe that Manhattan has four million rats until somebody asks YOU how they were counted.

On the subject of poop, you can ask a doctor about it. And you can ask a colon hygienist about it too. Doctors will tell you all sorts of things about poop and about colon hygiene, but you might investigate their record on slowing cases of colon cancer during the previous several decades.

As a colon hygienist I can tell you what I saw after cleansing my colon one hundred times and five hundred times and a thousand times. It's been quite interesting, not unlike a journey to the center of the earth. Strange creatures reside in the colon and it's worth writing a book about it.

Read what I have to say and arm yourself with the right questions. If you are an advanced student, you won't believe one word I say.

You will formulate your own mental models.

The sociology of poop

There are two sides to medicine. On the one hand, we witness brilliant success while on the other, miserable failures. When utilizing medicine, it would make sense to stay within the areas of brilliant success.

One way of doing this is to track the success rate of medicine over the past fifty years. Certain illnesses have been eliminated. Three cheers for medical research!

The failures of medicine include its job of preventing cancer, heart disease, obesity, and diabetes. Diseases of the colon have gone through the roof during our lifetime. It would be unwise to trust medicine to improve your odds in these areas, wouldn't it?

If the mental models of medicine have allowed diseases of the colon to skyrocket, then the basic mental models within medicine must be replaced. If medical researchers and doctors refuse to do this, then something is wrong. They are beating their heads against a wall and therefore if you go to them, you are beating your head against a wall.

Speaking as a colon hygienist, medicine gets it wrong by assuming the typical American's colon is basically clean. However, if you factor that our colons have become extremely toxic over the past fifty years, then other pieces of the health puzzle begin to make sense. The growing disease statistics fall into a reasonable explanation.

"If the mental models of medicine have allowed diseases of the colon to skyrocket, then the basic mental models within medicine must be replaced."

A researcher will never find the causes of colon diseases by looking through a microscope because they've been doing this for fifty years while these illnesses have only gotten worse. A sociologist has a better chance of showing cultural reasons for various diseases, if only given the chance to be included in the process.

A colon hygienist is a type of researcher too. When medicine begins looking outside of itself for answers, like to sociologists, environmentalists, and colon hygienists, perhaps real progress can be won.

Then we can all shout -- Go team! Go! Fight! *Win!*

Quacks and some crazy conclusions

The field of alternative healing has its own successes and its failures. People continue seeing quacks with as much enthusiasm as they visit doctors who have miserable track records.

How does one identify a quack?

Well, I spotted one the other day. If I tell you about my experience, perhaps it will help.

I attended a raw fooder's potluck with about 25 people attending. This is a group of folks interested in health through the means of a better diet. Each monthly get-together features a speaker on a health topic.

After everyone had eaten, a woman announced that she would be discussing the use of a pendulum. She began by saying that many of her friends and family thought her to be a quack. This is the first sign that a person is a quack. They generally identify themselves as one. See how simple it is!

She showed us a fat notebook filled with pictures of illnesses and lists of toxic chemicals. Using a swinging pendulum, she explained that her quackery was checking to see whether a client possessed any of the diseases or toxins in their body. I suppose she would then suggest natural therapies to correct and overcome the negative condition. No doubt pendulums have enthusiastic supporters who can trace their healing to its use.

She began testing everything around her -- a cup of water, a cell phone, food on a plate, and then moved to test the basic vitality of those in the room, including me. I couldn't see her pendulum because it was behind my back, but I heard her say, "See how the pendulum hangs -- this is an example of **low vitality**."

Then she asked me, "Are you eating a mostly raw diet?"

I replied, "My diet is actually very healthy."

Then she asked me to turn around and she gave me a treatment that included rubbing her hands down my spine and sweeping at my sacrum. Then she retested "my vitality" and demonstrated that it "had returned."

Next she tested the gentleman sitting next to me and found that he also had lost his vitality. She gave him the same basic treatment, except his vitality had returned with greater gusto than mine had. This she explained was due to the fact that he "probably had a better diet" which rendered him to respond quicker. Then she moved on.

Now -- a quick assessment:

#1) Beware the healer whose primary emphasis is **diagnosis**. You can pretty much count on the fact that they are a bearer of bad news.

#2) Beware the healer whose primary tool is a notebook filled with pictures of ugly diseases. Remember -- that which you focus upon, you attract. This woman mentioned that she herself had cancer at least three times, as recently as three months ago. A better form of service would be to fill a notebook with pictures of wonderful circumstances and use a pendulum to see which of these a person would want to attract.

#3) Beware the healers who have been repeatedly ill. On a psychic level they have something to prove. How much better to have nothing to prove and just be healthy.

#4) Beware the healer who would demonstrate "low vitality" to a room full of people without any personal intake. This is a basic slap across the face with the cooperation of other people in the room forming an agreement that "this person is less than well." Had I not been in a place of strength, this alone could have weakened my basic self image and immunity to negativity.

"Beware the healer whose primary emphasis is diagnosis."

However, this woman had no idea that her opinion had no power over me. The fact that she gave me "a diagnosis" of low vitality meant that she had absolutely no grasp of the power of her words and images before a group. She could have left me hanging.

Interesting to note that following the meeting, I conducted my own test. I milled around the room taking a reading of other people's attitudes toward me. To my amazement, people averted their eyes from me.

I had brought a cookbook titled, "Recipes for Life from God's Garden" by Rhonda Malkmus and had laid it on a table. As I went to pick it up, two people were standing by it commenting on it. One said, "That looks interesting," as I walked up.

As I reached for it, they recoiled. One said to the other, "It has recipes in it for *cooked* food," like this cookbook might be the source of my "low vitality."

#5) Beware the healer who brings a heavy spirit of criticism. Many healers think they are doing the world a great service when they awaken people's suspicions. BE SUSPICIOUS -- of the water. BE SUSPICIOUS -- of your food. BE SUSPICIOUS -- of the government. BE SUSPICIOUS -- of your neighbor.

The alternative is to bless your water, your food, your neighbor.

Allow me to point out that "being suspicious" has low power to birth positive change. An effective healer encourages others to OVERCOME negative circumstances, not just label and point them out to others. Finger pointing serves a role, but never mistake it for a healing energy in and of itself.

#6) Beware the healer who makes snap judgments with little or no information. When this woman stated that the gentleman sitting next to me had a better diet, she had nothing to base this upon. In fact, he had just told me his diet was far from perfect.

There are many, many components that make up a person's vitality and diet is just one of them. Her corrective measure of back-rubbing had absolutely **no relation** to diet. That's like going to the basement to fix a hole in the roof. If she was demonstrating low pendulum swing due to diet, the correction should be dietary in nature, such as drinking a shot of wheat grass, not back rubbing. Ask -- "Is this healer's basic logic sound?" I could have confronted her, but didn't think it was the time or place.

#7) Again, beware the healers who are not well themselves. Overcoming cancer naturally is not really a great thing for a healer's resume, especially repeated cases of cancer. Prevention means avoiding sickness in the first place.

#8) The final test of a quack is whether they give you new and heavy burdens to carry. Is their magic based upon removing the very burden they just handed to you? If so, thank the quack for his or her time and run in the opposite direction.

A true healer can say with a straight face that they are well. Ask a potential healer if they are well and how long they have been well. And then his or her goal should be to support *your* idea that you desire wellness.

If you sense that he or she has no interest in you as a complex human being, suspect that they have something up their sleeves. Bless them -- even confront them if it feels appropriate. But don't get into long arguments because that's the main damage quackery inflicts. It eats up your valuable time and energies.

How to find a reputable colonic therapist

Let's say you do your homework and your conclusion is that colonics might be a good thing for you to try. How do you find a reputable therapist?

First, they should not sell a lot of products. I recommend three basic products for colon health. 1) A quality probiotic which you can purchase at a health foods store or on the Internet for about $10. 2) A quality flax oil which you can purchase at a health food store or on the Internet for about $10. 3) A quality colon cleanser. There are lots of products that do this job, but avoid products containing psyllium.

If your colon hygienist sells other products, take down a list of what they suggest and compare prices on the Internet. If they sell "implants" at an extra charge, I'd suggest that it is a frill you don't need. If it is a wheat grass implant, you can usually get wheat grass at a health food store that you can drink orally with equal benefit. If it is a probiotic implant, you can receive just as much benefit from taking it orally. If your colon hygienist does not agree with me on implants, ask them if they believe in their position strongly enough to add it to your colonic session for no extra charge.

If your colon hygienist is assisting you because you have Candida yeast overgrowth, be cautious buying a lot of products too. Go online or buy them at your local health food store. Unless you are extremely motivated to kill Candida, understand that it is a long process that involves regular colon cleansing, establishing flora in the gut, and adding essential oil like flax to your diet. I realize I wrote earlier that a person can take a pill to treat yeast overgrowth, but I wasn't totally addressing the condition.

If you have chronic yeast infections, then I encourage you to conduct your own research, not just buy products. Ask for customer references. Surely he or she has two or three enthusiastic clients with goals similar to yours.

Secondly, your colon hygienist should be flushing your colon for at least thirty minutes, never shorter. That means your therapist is with you at least 45 minutes. If your therapist thinks they can clean your colon in under thirty minutes, find another therapist. If they want to argue this point, find another therapist.

I had one client coming from another colon hygienist who told me he received ten minute colonics. His therapist told him that his fecal matter came out so quickly that he finished early. No -- the therapist finished early, not the client!

"Your colon hygienist should be flushing your colon for at least thirty minutes, never shorter."

Thirdly, a long list of awards and credentials of the therapist means nothing in colon hygiene compared to having a basically good heart. Find someone who listens to and respects *you*.

Lastly, your therapist should encourage you to research and cleanse on your own without them. You can acquire an enema bag from your local drug store or buy some kind of home colonics unit from the Internet. Ultimately a colon hygienist's goal should be to train you and work themselves out of the job of keeping you internally clean.

Your ultimate realization -- you need more colonics than you should pay someone to give to you. Your therapist often just gets you started. Unless you are an exceptional case, internal cleansing can be done at home. A good colon hygienist blesses you as you ride off into the sunset.

Have fun getting clean

Some of my clients have been seeing me for years. For many it is not practical to install their own colonics unit at home. The reason I stated that a good colon hygienist should encourage you to cleanse on your own is because you should be aware that some therapists make their clients dependent on them and earn their living by selling expensive packages. But this can happen with any type of therapist or doctor.

Colon hygiene at first might present itself as a subject shrouded in mystery. If there is a colon hygienist office near you, go for one session and see what you think. The goal is very simple, to assist your body to remove fecal matter.

My client, David, called me last night to announce that his colema board was working great and he was seeing long ropes of fecal matter and slime coming out. I gave him the colema board for free and he is giving colema treatments to his girlfriend and she also experiences wonderful benefits. I suppose I lost their business, but I feel better knowing that there are two people on the planet better off for having met me.

It has been a couple of weeks since I wrote the above about David and he just phoned me again. He told me he has been taking bentonite clay, a super fine powder, along with his colema cleansing. He said that one tablespoon of clay has "the surface area of a football field" which absorbs impurities in the digestive tract. Within the past 30 hours, David said he had removed at least twenty-five feet of white gel-like ropes during two sessions. They came out in many foot-long sections before breaking off.

David had a colonoscopy ten months ago. I asked him if any observation had been made of such ropes in his colon during his colonoscopy. He said, no. I asked him if the laxative he had been given to drink before his colonoscopy had removed twenty-five feet of ropes. He said, no. I asked him if the ropes seemed like they had formed recently and he said, no, they smelled putrid and old.

A concern about colonics frequently mentioned to me is that water flushes the colon of valuable electrolytes. My opinion is that a putrid, septic colon has so many toxic substances that whatever beneficial substances are supposed to be inside the colon have been overcome by rot. I feel the same about beneficial bacteria inside a toxic colon. They have already been decimated. Colon cleaning clears the decimation out.

Many of David's friends and co-workers are asking what he has been doing because his appearance has dramatically improved. That does not happen when you are basically toxic and ill. People notice when you become more vibrant and energetic.

"Have fun getting clean. No matter what, it's always the same simple goal."

Another client recently teamed up with a friend who is a bit of a mad inventor. Without my help, he built his own colonics unit based on observing how mine worked. Again, I lost business on that, but have encouraged their independence.

The other day I drove to the guy's house to see his homespun unit and laughed at the ingenious design. He had installed a toilet float in his water tank so that it was self-filling at the perfect, constant temperature. Because the tank had to be installed quite high, he set his massage table on blocks so the height was about chest high. My client was in the process of giving herself a colonic and she looked like the "bride of Frankenstein" laying on a mad scientist's table. Totally cracked me up.

Have fun getting clean. No matter what, it's always the same simple goal. Get out the unwanted crap!

Debunking other common mental models

I went to lunch with a good friend and the subject of colonics came up. She told me she was afraid there might be horrible and nasty slime inside of her and she would rather not know. From my experience, every time I watched such foul stuff leave my body I felt nothing less than gratitude.

I've even talked to it saying, "See ya later, Slimy."

Once you get it out, it's gone. It ain't coming back. For me personally I'd rather know it's gone than to fear that it might be there and leave it inside.

It's not, "Hello, Slime."

It's, "Bye-bye, Slime."

A new client phoned me while I was at the grocery store. I said, "Hello," and immediately I was held captive by a woman on the other end talking about her thousand-and-one symptoms and every cure she had ever tried. If this was how she talked to me, imagine how she talked to herself! Finally, I had to cut her off.

"Excuse me," I said, "But that's more information than I'll need to know."

Silence.

Then she asked me, "How will you know what's wrong with me?"

"I don't need to know," I replied. "In fact, it is illegal for me to treat any kind of illness." Times like those I love the A.M.A.!

More silence on her end. This person had been trained to get all excited about her symptoms and then receive a dose of excitement back for how "whatever treatment" was going to help her amazingly. It completely threw her that I wasn't playing along.

"How would you want me to tell you that I was having a problem?" she asked.

"Don't tell me," I said abruptly. For some reason I was feeling bugged and recalled simpler times when you didn't carry a phone with you into a grocery store. Believe it or not, she made an appointment.

When she came in, I found her delightful, very well read, and knowledgeable about alternative health. She thanked me for helping her notice how much energy she was putting into her symptoms and made two more appointments.

When she phoned to make her third appointment I was again at the store and she was back to running at the mouth about her aches and pains and trying ever so hard to figure everything out with her brain. I told her, "You are still investing a huge amount of energy into your symptoms."

We didn't discuss much else over the phone and I was feeling like perhaps I needed to shift my career to writing instead of working with clients. *My* energy was shifting.

But then she brought me flowers she had picked from her garden, "To say, 'Thank you,'" she explained, "For the reminder to stop energizing symptoms."

Her thoughtfulness blessed me and also served to remind me not to take my cell phone into the grocery store. My annoyance was becoming my client's new therapy.

"She thanked me for helping her notice how much energy she was putting into her symptoms and made two more appointments."

The "more-war" on drugs

"I thought of medications as pretty much idiot-proof. You take them assuming that the worst that can happen is that they won't work. It turns out that the *worst* that can happen is that you drop dead. The next worse is that your body is permanently damaged. Less worse is that you suffer with something your doctor may or may not recognize as a drug reaction -- anything from a skin rash to heart failure to a sudden inability to have an orgasm. Your doctor may mistake it for another illness and give you more drugs for that, leading to the so-called 'cascade of prescribing.'"

--Stephen Fried, *Bitter Pills*

A middle-aged client came to me who is a doctor. He works at an emergency room. Without any prompting from me he said, "I've observed that the patients who take the most medications are the most ill."

I replied with a question: "Do you think those who are the most ill are taking so many medications because they are ill and need the drugs?"

"People in the emergency room often ask for drugs by name."

He didn't reply immediately, but I could tell he had already considered that. "No," he replied, "I don't think so."

"You think it's the other way around?"

It felt like he was confessing something to me without really confessing anything, but he said, "Yeah, I think it's the other way around."

In other words, the medications come first and a lowered vitality comes second. He told me about a recent patient who was age 96 and was brought to the emergency room by his daughter. "That guy was taking no medications and you could tell he was still basically very healthy," the doctor mused.

He also told me that people in the emergency room often ask for drugs by name before he has even given them an examination. He said, "It's out of control."

"What do you do?" I asked.

"I usually write them a prescription," he replied. "People don't feel like they've been successfully treated these days unless they leave with a prescription."

Chapter Seven
Pay Attention

"I found about 60 or 70 different case studies showing that virtually every prescription medicine we take depletes the body of a nutrient. I can only think of a handful of people throughout the country even thinking about this. I can't begin to describe to you the acceleration of disease and what is happening to the American public."

-- Dr. Derrick DeSilva, M.D., on staff at the John F. Kennedy Medical Center

Among the worst offenders of nutrient depletion are the cholesterol-lowering drugs known as statins.

In the bestseller, *The South Beach Diet*, readers over age forty are encouraged to begin taking these drugs along with aspirin. Not mentioned, however, is the proven fact that statin drugs deplete the body of coenzyme Q10.

"If you're taking a statin drug you must, and I repeat you must, be giving your body coenzyme Q10."

What does CoQ10 do for the body? Dr. Robert Atkins writes in his book, *Vita-Nutrient Solution*, that CoQ10 is "absolutely vital to our health, essential to energy production in our every cell, allowing the cells to live much longer."

Contrast the depletion of this nutrient with the pharmaceutical industry pushing statin drugs on younger Americans, even for adolescents with a family history of heart disease. According to Dr. DeSilva, "It is very, very, very well known that the statin drugs deplete the body of coenzyme Q10. If you're taking a statin drug you must, and I repeat you must, be giving your body coenzyme Q10. I'm not saying get off your drugs. What I'm saying is take the appropriate nutrients with them."

When a doctor says "very" three times in a row, I think that means he wants you to listen very, very, very closely. And my client, Roy, will be pleased to see that I am quoting from a medically trained professional.

Nuclear effects of a microwave oven

"The whole world is governed by a pulsation, connected with the planets and much more beyond."
Alan Chadwick, *Villa Montalvo Lecture Series*

Our physical bodies and our spirits are affected by subtle energies that are now detected by the most sensitive scientific instruments. Electromagnetic devices upon which humanity depends are everywhere and their impact on general well-being -- our physical bodies -- cannot be calculated.

Take the microwave oven. Most mothers and fathers today wouldn't think twice about the subtle changes microwave heating causes to the food they prepare. It's become a uniquely American cooking tradition for over a quarter of a century.

However, Russian scientists have conducted investigations into microwave heating which were published by the Atlantis Raising Educational Center in Portland, Oregon. Here is a partial summary of their tests:

- Microwaving prepared meats sufficiently to insure sanitary ingestion caused formation of d-Nitrosodienthanolamines, a well-known carcinogen.
- Microwaving milk and cereal grains converted some of their amino acids into carcinogens (cancer-causing substances).
- Thawing frozen fruits converted their glucoside and galactoside-containing fractions into carcinogenic substances.
- Extremely short exposure of raw, cooked, or frozen vegetables converted their plant alkaloids into carcinogens.

- Carcinogenic free radicals were formed in microwaved plants, especially root vegetables.

Sources: *Well Being Journal* Winter 2001 and *Health & Wellness* by Patricia Martin. Nov.-Dec. 2000.

Swiss biologist, Dr. Hans Hertel, studied the effects of eating microwaved food, published in *Nexus Magazine.* Overall, the study suggested that eating microwaved foods can cause degenerative illness. Microwaves heat by "reversing polarity" and this tears and deforms molecular structure, creating new compounds not found in nature called "radiolytic compounds." In simple terms, useful life-force is dissipated by 60 to 90 percent. Eating microwaved food, over time, causes significant negative changes in blood chemistry.

Research this on the Internet under "Microwave and health and danger."

At the very least, never microwave food in a plastic tray or under plastic wrap. If you must microwave, use glass dishes only. I owned the same microwave oven since college. It was like my little buddy, but as soon as I learned about the potential effects of its radiation, I thanked it for its years of service and heaved it into the dumpster.

"Eating microwaved foods can cause degenerative illness."

Liver detox and weight loss

Excerpt from *First for Women* by Brenda Kearns

"'An overburdened liver is the #1 weight-loss stumbling block and fatigue trigger from women (and men), and the one factor that can foil even the most determined dieter,' says naturopath Linda Page, N.D., Ph.D., the country's foremost authority on nutritional healing. And it's not surprising that this football-sized organ is prone to exhaustion: it's responsible for more than 1,500 metabolic reactions (many of them essential for proper fat-burning and energy production) and serves as a vast nutrient storehouse.

'When environmental pollutants, a poor diet or any other factor overburdens the liver, it becomes less efficient at burning body fat and converting food to energy,' says Dr. Page. 'In fact, by her 20th birthday, almost every woman has some degree of liver exhaustion, and a sluggish liver means a sluggish you,' she says.

But now there's good news: Your liver can actually regenerate itself if it's properly cleansed and detoxified -- virtually erasing fatigue and speeding up weight loss. Liver cleansing flushes fat from the stomach, buttocks and thighs."

"Your liver can actually regenerate itself if it's properly cleansed and detoxified."

There are many recipes for a detoxification of the liver. However, most Americans are so backed up that they can't pass what is removed from the liver before the body recycles the bile fluid. Therefore, if you plan to do any sort of liver cleanse, prepare the way by doing colonics both before and after the cleanse.

Margarine -- who's still buying it?
(And are they *crazy?*)

Partially-hydrogenated oils are some of the most *alien* substances modern food processing has introduced into the diet -- and it's frequently found in packaged foods from bakery items to pasta sauce. The simplest way to avoid it is to begin reading the ingredients listed on food labels. It is also known as margarine.

It's listed right on the label: *partially-hydrogenated oil.* It is a "transfat."

Healthy Fats For Life, written by Lorna R. Vanderhaeghe and Karlene Karst, states: "Numerous research studies have shown that transfats are more damaging to the heart than saturated fats, and, in fact, ... there are no safe levels of transfats and the consumption should be reduced as much as possible. They are man made, formed by a process of high temperature and hydrogenation that turns refined oils into margarines, shortenings and partially hydrogenated vegetable oils. Our bodies cannot recognize them as nutrients and therefore are not able to process them. They are, however, a food manufacturer's dream as they are inexpensive to produce and extend the shelf life of foods. The Harvard School of Public Health has declared transfats dangerous to our health." (Page 4.)

Animal fat, such as butter, has been blamed for our nation's epidemic of heart disease. However, from 1920 through 1989, animal fat consumption declined from 25 pounds to 10.5 pounds per capita. Vegetable fats increased during that same time from 10 pounds to 50.4 pounds per capita, a 500-percent increase.

Could partially-hydrogenated vegetable oils found in most every form of processed food be the real culprit contributing to heart disease? Almost half of the packaged products you see at the grocery store contain transfats, including products labeled as "low fat." Most cookies, cake mixes, frozen breakfast foods, snacks and chips, and even breakfast cereals, contain partially-hydrogenated oils.

"Almost half of the packaged products you see at the grocery store contain transfats, including products labeled as low fat."

Like the authors of *Healthy Fats For Life,* you should ask, "Are transfats really that bad? The simple answer -- they are deadly." Here is a partial list of some of the chapter titles from this book describing the importance of quality oils (EFAs) in the diet:

- Win the War Against Weight
- Type 2 Diabetes: You May Be at Risk
- Heart Health: Have a Love Affair with Fat
- Boost Your Brain, Improve Mental Health
- Healthy Fats, Healthy Hormones
- The Diet and Breast Cancer Link

- Optimal Oils for Bones and Joints
- Prostate Protection

As far as the colon goes, anything that impairs function of any of the organs, impairs the digestive, assimilation, and elimination processes. The best book I have read on the topic of essential fats is called, "Fats that Heal, Fats that Kill," by Udo Erasmus. If you only read one book about health during your lifetime, that should be it. Mr. Erasmus also has a web site: www.udoerasmus.com.

A green mustache is a better sign of calcium intake

"The Federal Trade Commission in April, 1974, issued a 'proposed complaint' against the California Milk Producers Advisory Board and their advertising agency. In this complaint they cited the slogan 'Everybody Needs Milk' as representing false, misleading, and deceptive advertising. The FTC judged that enthusiastic testimonials ... conveyed an inaccurate picture of the value of milk as food. Quickly the dairymen changed their approach and came up with a new slogan: 'Milk has Something for Everybody.' This is certainly technically correct. The question you must ask yourself before you drink that next glass of milk, however, is: do you really want that 'something?'"
-- Frank A. Oski, M.D., *Don't Drink Your Milk!*

Milk has been touted to build strong bones. How can this be? Americans have the highest levels of osteoporosis while consuming more dairy products than other nations. Today we eat about 30 lbs. of cheese annually, nearly double since the 1950s.

One reason dairy can harm us is because the human body requires a specific blood pH that is continually balanced. A diet high in proteins (such as with The Atkin's Diet) **forms <u>acids</u>** in the body that must be neutralized. Americans are eating mostly acid-forming foods and this causes alkalines (calcium) to be leached from the bones.

If you eat food that is more acidic than your blood, then how will the blood balance itself? It has one option: draw from stores of alkalines making up bones.

"A diet high in proteins (such as with The Atkin's Diet) forms acids in the body that must be neutralized."

In addition, supplementing calcium won't help because a deficiency of intestinal flora prevents its absorption. Aftab J. Ahmed, Ph.D., concurs with this in his article, *Osteoporosis: Diet, Acidity and Calcium.* He writes, "Absorption of calcium can be maximized by jump-starting proliferation of colonic flora ... an optimally functional GI system ensures a requisite supply." Intestinal flora help condition the colon's lining such that minerals can be diffused through the digestive tract into the blood.

Another reason is that insufficient bile production causes fats in dairy products to bond with calcium which further prevents its absorption into the bloodstream.

Milk alone would not, and *could* not, improve calcium absorption nor prevent osteoporosis caused from an acid-forming diet and from deficiencies in intestinal flora.

Another issue with milk: One of my clients, Frances, came for a colonic weekly and each time she released about two feet of translucent mucus. It came out in foot-long sections resembling a sugar cone, like a brown ice cream cone made from rubber. I saw this with such regularity that I never thought to question it until one day she happened to mention that she drank a lot of milk.

Suddenly it became obvious. We correlated the milk to the mucus we saw during her colonics. After she cut back on drinking milk, the mucus immediately vanished.

I keep organic milk in the refrigerator, but don't drink it. Perhaps it's nostalgia from when I was a kid. Other than that, my daughter likes milk on her cereal. I have nothing against cows and dairy farmers and hope that we all stay healthy for a long time.

Consuming green, leafy kale is the ideal source of calcium all the way around. In other words, the color of your mustache should be green, same as cows should have.

Here comes the sun

On a sunny, hot day I saw a couple driving in a convertible and something looked out of place. Both people wore hats with visors, sun glasses, long sleeve shirts, and rode slumped down in their seats like they were traveling incognito. Then it struck me what they were hiding from -- the sun!

This past summer I attended a family reunion held at the beach. It was astounding to observe the amounts of sun screen folks were gobbing all over their largest bodily organ, the skin. Their concern had nothing to do with the list of ingredients making up the lotion, but only with "the number" printed on the bottle. I personally avoid sun screen so I don't have a high interest in the ingredients either.

I love the sun. Having lived in Alaska for nine years, I appreciate feeling the heat of the sun's rays as much as I can. I consider there's not much finer than to spend an afternoon outside shirtless. If I am by the ocean or at a lake, I WANT to absorb the natural waters into my skin. How can that happen if my skin is coated in an unnatural film of waterproof "protective" sunscreen?

Something most people would never consider is the toxicity of chemicals they put onto their skin in combination, like sun screen with mosquito repellent or sun screen with women's face make-up. If incidence of skin cancer is at record highs, maybe this American obsession with sun lotion is misplaced. Perhaps it isn't protecting us. Perhaps we are *over*protecting ourselves.

The following is a quote from Tonya Zavasta's book, *Your Right to be BEAUTIFUL: How to halt the train of aging and meet the most beautiful you.* I consider these two paragraphs to offer everything you need to know about "the sun and you."

"David Wolf, in his book, *Sunfood Diet,* writes that the human body draws in sunlight with many capillaries on the skin surface, and the blood's hemoglobin converts it directly into nourishment, just as chlorophyll converts sunlight into nourishment in plants. He suggests that the same substances which protect leaves from ultra-violet radiation in green-leafed vegetables by shielding the nucleus of each cell, will also protect us when we ingest those leaves."

"On the other hand, a diet high in cooked fat and processed foods has been linked to skin cancer. When the body is polluted with metabolic and chemical waste, too many toxins get pushed out through the skin ... fried and mutated when exposed to the sun's rays. Blaming nature for skin problems, instead of our own actions, is absurd. After several years on the (Raw) diet, the sun will no longer threaten your skin."

"A diet high in cooked fat and processed foods has been linked to skin cancer."

For more information, go to www.BeautifulOnRaw.com.

By the way, the morning sun contains the element lithium, which when taken into the human body elevates mood naturally.

Inside poop on artificial sweeteners

What is aspartame? Ask me again and I'll tell you the same. Here's more from Tonya Zavasta. I thank her for permission to include her research. Basically -- her findings can't be improved upon, so why pretend? I'd tell you the same.

"The more artificial sweeteners you consume, the more likely you are to actually gain weight."

"Implications of cancer, even though clearly serious, are not the only problem with artificial sweeteners. These substances are used mainly for their low calorie content ... and are much sweeter than sugar ... aspartame being 200 times as sweet as sugar ... and Sweet

'N Low ten times sweeter. When artificial sweeteners are consumed, the brain registers the intense sweetness and prepares the intestinal tract for an enormous intake of calories that does not arrive with the low calorie sweetener. The body will produce enzymes to convert **future calories** to fat."

"According to Stephen Cherniske in *Caffeine Blues*, when you consume a diet soft drink, even though the beverage contains only one calorie, your body becomes prone to create fat as soon as you eat some real food. That's why, the more artificial sweeteners you consume, the more likely you are to actually gain weight. This is confirmed by a study conducted on 80,000 women over a period of six years as reported in a 1986 issue of *Preventative Medicine*."

Taken from Tonya's book, *Your Right to be BEAUTIFUL.*

More on sweetener

Many of us consume more than our body weight in added sugar and sweeteners every year. The per capita average was 152 pounds in 2000, up 11 percent from 1990. Of course, if graphed over the past century, sugar consumption has climbed year after year after year like a jet after take-off.

My nineteen year-old son, Art, started getting acne on his face over night. I was reading Tonya Zavasta's book and came across the theory that sugar can be a significant cause of acne. Despite my respect for the author, I initially scoffed at the idea.

I decided to ask Art: "Has your sugar intake increased recently?"

My question stopped him in his tracks. He replied with one word, "Yes," in such a way that it implied, "How did you know?"

He was working at a new job as a busboy and all the staff had free access to the Coke machine. He said everybody drank Coke like it was going out of style. It kept everybody buzzed and hopping, he said.

We tried a little experiment. He switched from cola to bottled water. His acne disappeared as quickly as it had appeared.

Thing is, this solution did not come from my logic or from my reasoning ability. The odds of timing were at least 1000:1 that I would read about sugar's role in causing acne at the exact same moment that my son got pimples. If I had read about it before his acne appeared, I wouldn't have remembered this information because I had such serious doubts about it even as I skimmed over it.

I had, however, pictured my son well, which made all the difference.

Why you don't want to be an old salt

Yes, *more* from Tonya. And I'd still tell you the same ... there's no improvement required here because she makes it perfectly clear.

"Three thousand years ago, salt was still a rare commodity. When it was discovered that salt had the magical property of preserving food, the human obsession with salt began. The National Academy of Sciences recommends consumption of a minimum of 500 milligrams a day of sodium to maintain good health. The majority of Americans consume seven to 10 times more."

"In the 1950s, physicians began to advise people to take salt tablets during hot weather as a replacement for sodium lost during perspiration. In the 1980s, the medical profession made a U-turn in its opinion and advised Americans to eliminate or reduce salt intake to avoid high blood pressure. Recent research suggests that a low-salt diet has minimal effect on blood pressure. So the doctor's advice has been swinging like a pendulum. The reason for this woeful contradiction is that organic sodium is equated with the inorganic component of sodium chloride."

"The terms 'salt' and 'sodium' are often used interchangeably, but this is not correct. When table salt is dissolved it breaks down into two components: positively charged sodium (metal) and negatively charged chlorine (gas). Chemically, this sodium is the same as the sodium derived from an organic source, but there is a fundamental difference in its action on the body. A low-sodium diet cuts down on the intake of inorganic sodium, which is good, but it also calls for avoiding organic sources of sodium, which is dangerous."

"Doctor's advice has been swinging like a pendulum."

"While medical experts appear to be hopelessly confused about salt, all beauty experts agree unanimously: Salt makes you look puffy. The human body cannot survive without sodium, but it will do beautifully without table salt. When a particle of (table) salt enters the body, it is recognized as a foreign substance, a poison, and the body acts to defend itself. In an attempt to protect the surrounding cells from this highly irritating substance, the body will retain water. According to *Salt Conspiracy*, by Victoria Bidwell, one ounce of ingested salt retains 3 quarts of water, which translates into 6 pounds of excess body water and fluids in suspension."

"Sodium chloride is a toxic, inorganic compound, unusable by the body, that leads to premature aging and degenerative diseases. Dr. Max Gerson treated terminally ill cancer patients with a highly nutritious diet. According to his research, the beginning of all chronic disease is the loss of potassium from the cells and the invasion of sodium into the cells. Sodium does not cause cancer, but it is always a major player. In his book, *A Cancer Therapy: Results of Fifty Cases and the Cure of Advanced Cancer,* he states that by removing excess sodium from the body, the edema that protects the malignant cells can also be eliminated. Then the way is provided for oxygen and enzymes from fresh raw vegetables and juices to attack the cancer cells."

"During the last two centuries, the increased use of preservatives has altered the taste buds of many people, making them addicted to the taste of salt. If we eat processed food, we get additional sodium and not enough potassium. Surrounding cells lose their water to dilute the briny intercellular fluid. The space between the cells swells while the cells and capillaries lose potassium and become dehydrated. Capillaries begin to constrict and lose elasticity. Salt intake will shrink, calcify, and scar the muscles and arteries. The greatest offender in the use of salt is the food processing industry."

Taken from *Your Right to be BEAUTIFUL,* by Tonya Zavasta. For more information, go to www.BeautifulOnRaw.com.

Is your fluoridated water safe?

Provided by Daniel M. Stockin, Senior Operations Officer
The Lillie Center, Inc.

For more than 50 years, most Americans have believed that adding fluoride to water and toothpaste is safe, effective, and necessary for the prevention of cavities. Now, information pouring in from around the world is showing that ingested fluoride is causing or contributing to many conditions we've come to expect as "diseases of aging." Included are hip fractures, thyroid disease, and joint pain, as well as several other disorders that affect persons of all ages.

It has now come out that most of the fluoride we've been injecting into our drinking water is a type of silicofluoride, a substance that has never been tested or approved by any federal agency. Where does it come from? It is an air pollutant emission captured by smokestack "scrubber" equipment at phosphate fertilizer factories! If it is emitted into the air, it is a pollutant; if it is discharged into a lake or river, it is a pollutant; it is regulated by EPA as a water "contaminant;" but if it is placed in our drinking water and we ingest it into our bodies, it has somehow been deemed a "nutrient." Because of the industrial processes and raw material used as its source, the fluoride also comes contaminated with radioactive compounds, arsenic, lead, and mercury.

Why weren't we told this? Well, we were ... but not really. Buried in many water agencies' water quality reports amongst a dizzying list of chemical names has been a little-observed statement that the source of the fluoride is "discharge from fertilizer and aluminum factories." Those who thought to ask about it have been told that the toxic fluoride, arsenic, and radioactive compounds are diluted in the water, therefore they pose no harm. But what is usually not said is that these compounds are cumulative poisons. The small amounts we ingest daily cumulatively build up in our bodies and can cause cancer, thyroid disease, kidney damage, and joint pain.

Some of these diseases also have side effects, such as the weight gain and depression of thyroid disease. How do you feel that your body is being used as the final resting place of the toxic discharges of industry?

"What is usually not said is that these compounds are cumulative poisons."

It also turns out that in 2000, dentists admitted that fluoride helps prevent cavities primarily topically, while in the mouth -- not by your body's systemic absorption of the chemical. So then the logical question is: why continue drinking a toxic chemical throughout your whole body, over your entire lifetime, if its main action against cavities occurs when it touches teeth in the mouth?

Did you or your children ever swallow toothpaste? Look on the back of your fluoridated toothpaste tube. It says that children swallowing fluoride may require calling a poison control center. You also receive fluoride in your foods -- in your cereal, bread, canned foods, tea, sodas, pasta, baby food, and frozen foods (because they're made with fluoridated water), as well as from antibiotics. Due to lack of investigation, education, and oversight, we have cumulatively been overdosing on a known poison that affects DNA, enzymes, and every organ system in the body.

You and your family should take steps to protect yourselves. If your water district fluoridates its water, urge your local authorities to stop fluoridating. Drink and cook only with unfluoridated water. Use a reverse osmosis or distillation unit to filter your home's water. Carbon filters do not remove fluoride. Use an unfluoridated toothpaste that you can find at health food stores. Do not give your children fluoride supplements. Educate yourself about the sources and harmful health effects of fluoride by visiting www.thelilliecenter.com or www.fluoridealert.org. Remember: despite what dentists have told us, fluoride is not safe, and there are plenty of other ways to prevent cavities, such as good oral hygiene and reducing the amount of sugars in your diet.

How to research health issues

Somebody asked me about what was causing so many gall bladder removal operations in America. I randomly picked up one of my book resources and opened it by coincidence at the page discussing the gall bladder. In other words, such a huge problem in America ... so easily understood and solved!

I quote from Brenda Watson's book, "Renew Your Life":

"Bile secretions is one of the liver's most important functions. Bile ... contains toxins that have been processed by chemical reactions (in the liver) to render them safe for elimination. The bile is stored temporarily in the gall bladder where water and minerals are reabsorbed making the bile more concentrated, which improves efficiency in digesting fat. .... and serves as a carrier medium for the elimination of many toxic substances from the body ... absorbed by dietary fiber and excreted."

"In the absence of fiber, the toxins are reabsorbed. Since bile is the carrier medium, diminished bile flow is a significant contributor to liver impairment. When excretion of bile is inhibited, toxins remain in the liver too long. As it stores more toxins, its efficiency is compromised, and bile flow decreases. Thus the liver can become constipated just like the colon."

"Another problem can occur when bile ducts become blocked, usually by gallstones ... thought to be from an imbalance of bile salts and minerals, dehydration, toxins and excess cholesterol in the bile. In addition, a high fat, low fiber diet has been associated with gall stone production. Gall stones can be a real medical problem, blocking the flow of bile from the liver and gall bladder and sometimes obstructing the pancreas and intestines as well. These situations often constitute a surgical emergency."

Traditional medicine would stop here. Doctors perform surgery to remove "the problem" and recommend a high fiber, low fat diet. End of story? Not at all.

Let's read on:

"Yet another common problem is the excretion of toxic bile (bile not chemically transformed adequately by the liver's enzyme system). Toxic bile can literally burn the bile ducts, the gall bladder, the intestines, eventually leading to hepatitis, cholecystitis, pancreatitis, and inflammation of the liver, gall bladder, pancreas and duodenum. Toxic bile could ultimately contribute to the development of cancer of the involved organs. Gall bladder problems then can develop when the liver is so overloaded that it sends toxins on to the gall bladder before neutralized. Irritation from these toxins can cause the gall bladder to malfunction."

SO -- if we flow-chart this process, we see that modern medicine has gone crazy with the removal of the gall bladder and totally ignores the SOURCE of inflammation -- toxic bile.

"Modern medicine has gone crazy with the removal of the gall bladder and totally ignores the SOURCE of inflammation."

Doctors may recommend <u>dietary</u> changes -- which are not based on reality.

1) Patients believe that the weak link is the organ itself and therefore will not correct their diet. 2) Most people refuse to change their diets anyway. 3) Even if they changed their diet to high fiber/ low fat, it would make ZERO difference, I repeat ZERO.

This is because the SOURCE of toxic bile has not been addressed -- i.e., from toxic food additives/chemicals and pharmaceutical toxins, etc., consumed daily. AND, if the gall bladder has become irritated enough to cause pain/symptoms, we know the colon is completely plugged because digesting food has had insufficient bile added over time -- and fats not properly digested create hard stools, further slowing transit time.

Fiber at this point only MAKES THINGS WORSE, like added gum. My clients who take fiber supplements have the worst constipation which forms a length of poop roughly five feet long held in the gut despite a daily bowel movement.

Plus, most toxic chemicals require oils to make them soluble enough to be eliminated, and Americans are not consuming these "right" oils because of fat phobia/ignorance. YET, even if a person ate more fiber and the right oils, it's too little too late -- because the colon is backed up already, slowing transit time so that chemical poisons are reabsorbed into the body before they can be eliminated.

THIS IS WHY COLONICS ARE NECESSARY and the best alternative to surgery, at the very least -- prevention.

Colon cleansing is the only way to increase transit time and allow toxin-removal today. The gall bladder's role is only one stage of the larger detox cycle.

The alternative approach is to study the flow chart of the CAUSES of toxic bile. On the front end this includes all sources of toxic man-made chemicals. If a person lessens the load here as prevention, the entire bodily system benefits.

On the back end, if you cleanse the colon from congestion, then you free the liver/gall bladder to dump poisons -- before they can be reabsorbed. If you surgically remove the gall bladder, it should be plain to see that nothing has been done to solve the creation of and the elimination of the toxic bile and another problem will eventually manifest. Without looking at the statistics, I would bet that another growing surgical procedure for females is the hysterectomy, while the original problem is toxic bile.

That said, how is it that my twenty minutes of research has made me an expert on gall bladder removal while today's doctors spend years in study and still suffer from surgical myopia? You tell me! In the macro-culture, everything we're told is upside-down. All across the board is a clouding of facts and "someone" benefits from the mass confusion.

The current situation -- a person goes to their doctor from symptoms associated with gall bladder dysfunction. The doctor knows that diet changes won't solve the problem fast enough -- so they remove the gall bladder. Yet we already know the source of the problem continues -- toxicity of bile, insufficiency of bile, and a congested colon. What happens next? For that we return to Brenda Watson.

She writes: "The liver metabolizes hormones, notably testosterone and estrogen. Poor liver function, coupled with deficiencies of good colonic bacteria, results in hormonal imbalances in both men and women that can put them at risk for developing serious disease."

What we have here is the connection between gall bladder

removal in women and related complications of estrogen toxicity. Removing the gall bladder does nothing to correct this issue, yet cleaning the colon ALSO ADDRESSES estrogen toxicity. In addition, a clean colon facilitates the growth of good bacteria, which in turn manufacture B vitamins, which in turn can be used by the liver to detoxify excess estrogen.

Surgery facilitates a downward health spiral and further surgery. Internal cleansing facilitates improved function of all internal organs and an upward health spiral.

So, what is happening on a mass scale? Watson continues: "Certain B vitamins are needed by the liver to detoxify estrogen and excrete it with the bile. With today's widespread vitamin B deficiencies, estrogen is not metabolized properly, and the result is increased levels of toxic estrogen metabolites. ... This diminishes bile flow, resulting in further reduction of estrogen detoxification and clearance. Conditions such as PMS, fibrocystic breast disease, ovarian cysts, uterine fibroids, and cancer of the breast, ovaries and uterus have been associated with elevated estrogen."

Like I suggested earlier, my guess is that the hysterectomy falls next on the list of surgeries for women following gall bladder removal. And breast cancer surgery. It's misguided -- impairing millions of patients who have various symptoms and making lots of doctors rich. If a patient questions their doctor why one surgery was only a temporary solution, the doctor brings up dietary factors -- not only does the patient feel guilty over their horrible diet, it relieves doctors from any responsibility that surgery breeds surgery.

Twenty minutes of research. Quiz yourself now to see what can be easily discovered flipping through information readily available.

What's at stake? Not much except possibly sparing yourself from unnecessary surgery, recovering your health, and maybe saving your life.

If you ever doubt your own findings, you can always consult your doctor.

Chapter Eight
Health benefits of enthusiasm

This morning a brand new client who never had a colonic climbed up on the table and told me about a friend of hers who refused to consider internal cleansing. She said, "I can't make him do it." How interesting to me that people can't get well alone. They need to bring others with them. I said to her, "Get over it -- save *yourself*!"

After her, I had a guy come who is doing fifteen colonics within three weeks. He raised the identical problem, that his wife had so many health problems and he just *wished* she would do some colon cleansing.

I told him that I had another client in the same boat with a close friend -- lots of unhealthy symptoms and terror at the mention of colonics. "What did you tell her?" he asked.

"I told her, 'Get over it -- save yourself,'" I replied.

He laughed, but seemed sad when he said, "I suppose you can't do anything for them then."

"No," I said, "There's *lots* you can do."

"Like what?"

"You can believe for them ..." I explained, "Hope for their best ... imagine them as healthy as a horse, happy, overjoyed! Always, always want the best for those you love, and that is doing a lot. To *want* something is a form of prayer."

"Always, always want the best for those you love."

I've had down moments myself where I thought, "Scott, you're going down with the ship."

Then I think -- "Wait a minute! Other people have risen from circumstances way worse than mine. I'm not handicapped except in the ways I handicap myself. This gallows is of my own making. This is America."

So I say to myself, "Go to bed. Get some sleep! Wake up in the morning and triple your efforts. Damn the torpedoes! Swab the deck. Raise the gang plank! Set sail. We're in the land of opportunity!"

There's lots we can say to ourselves other than, "Nobody's doing nothing and it's all going to pot." If things are that bad, make yourself a sign and go down to the corner to bum yourself some money to buy some fresh fruit that somebody else grew for you and sit outside under a tree and start counting your blessings starting with the letter "A".

A client said to me yesterday, "I feel so depressed about the world situation."

I said, "Has it done anybody any good?"

"What?"

"Your feeling depressed," I replied. "Who's it helped?"

Depressed people are actually easier to control. Everybody seems so worried about some governmental agency controlling our thoughts that "Big Brother" doesn't need to *bother*. How can we impact anything wrong the government might attempt while we lie on the couch feeling forlorn?

This one client told me how she worried about satellites watching her from space, telling me she can get a photo of her house's roof off the Internet. I said, "Good God! Do you really think George Bush cares about you so much that he's getting photo feeds of your daily activities? Like, 'Here she is leaving to go to the grocery store. There she is getting the mail.'"

If people prayed by feeling enthusiasm well-up into their spirits over some wonderful thing they were going to do that nobody ever dreamed possible, by golly, things will change. Have we forgotten? That's what built America.

Get excited, damn it!

"What is truly great is accessible to all." -- Soren Kierkegaard

My client, Frances, has come for a colonic almost weekly for four years. After about one year, I encouraged her to install a colonics unit in her home. I went to her house and we surveyed where we might put it.

Then she decided she didn't want to do it. Her reason was because she enjoyed coming to my office. It provided her a much needed break in her busy week.

One day she came to my office in tears. She worked for a communications company as a sales manager and her boss was constantly and unreasonably critical. While getting her colonic we discussed the ways she wanted to feel in her job -- appreciated, uplifted, enthusiastic. One benefit from a colonic is that the release of built-up fecal matter improves mental clarity and attitude and so she left her session noticeably much better in spirit.

"God works through miracles beyond our scope to invent."

The following week she still felt frustrated to overcome her feelings of loathing toward her boss. We discussed how to release her from the responsibility of changing her feelings because it seemed so difficult for her. Ultimately she surrendered her situation to God. I suggested she surrender each time she felt burdened because God carries our burdens. And God works through miracles beyond our scope to invent.

About one month later, she announced that her entire office was being closed by the corporate headquarters and *everybody* was losing their job. She said that she actually felt relief because she would soon be free of her terrible boss, even if it meant her own unemployment.

A week later she said that the company was maintaining a skeleton crew in Nashville and that she was on the list of those potentially keeping their job. It was not very long before she was given the unlikely opportunity to watch her boss pack his things and she made amends with him -- after he was gone. She sat in his empty office, in his very chair, and wished him well.

Her new boss was based in another state and was a perfect match in temperament for her working style. It wasn't long before she discovered someone else in the organization who held a position of power over her who rubbed her wrong. I said, "Frances, this repeat problem is obviously about you. As soon as you are able to love this sort of person, they will magically disappear."

This high level manager had singled her out during a meeting and had thrashed her performance in front of her peers on what she perceived to be minor matters. Now she was soon to give a presentation to a group of managers including him and she felt such resentment that she feared she would cry if he picked on her again. I encouraged her to send him love every time she thought of him.

When the meeting came around she did such a great job that this very manager praised her in front of the group and later phoned Frances personally to apologize for his previous bad behavior.

Then Frances had another problem. She had gotten a great deal on a new car, an off-brand model, but when she took it for a minor repair she was told it would take weeks to fix because parts were nearly impossible to find. She felt trapped in a car that was no longer imported into America. Strange as it sounds, we did a quick exercise where she imagined herself in a car she completely loved driving.

Hard as it might seem to believe, Frances was rear-ended at a traffic light and despite the minor damage, her insurance company totaled the car because new parts simply were not available. Suddenly she found herself in a new American-made car.

Is this magic? No, it's a natural law and a spiritual law.

The story continues. Frances then said she was beginning to feel out of sync with her primary customer. The staff was demanding and unappreciative, she explained.

"I believe we are going to see a change in your work very soon," I said.

She reviewed the job postings with her company and phoned human resources about a position as a trainer with new staff. Unfortunately she was told that the position had just been filled. A week later she received a call that the person hired changed her mind and the position was again posted. It previously was based in another city, but now it would be moved to Nashville. She interviewed and got the position, which turned out to be her dream job.

And the manager she once had trouble with, the guy she had practiced sending love, turned out to be instrumental in helping her change positions. In a double twist of fate, her old position was phased out after the primary customer did not renew the annual contract on the national level. I told Frances that if she had written a script of moves she needed to take to stay employed, she couldn't have maneuvered more perfectly. When a person surrenders to a Higher Love and Intelligence, powers are released beyond the imagination to work on their behalf.

It turned out that Frances was smart to come to my office each week for moral and spirit-related support. Two people's strategic optimism can accomplish a lot.

Another client came to me recently, Lynn, an actress. She is employed by the Grand Ol' Opry, but told me that she would soon be out of work. I took out my cell phone and began talking into it like I had just received a call: *"You want me to act for you? Am I available? Sure! How much did you say it pays? Wow! That's wonderful."*

I looked at her and asked, "Do you know what I am doing?"

"I have no idea," she replied.

"I'm suggesting that you demonstrate to the loving Universe that you are ready for your next job and that you are taking calls from people paying you great sums of money."

When Lynn came back for another colonic she announced that she had received two phone calls exactly like I had demonstrated. This could seem coincidental, but the next bit of detail is beyond coincidence.

I bumped into Lynn's friends who had referred her to my services and since I hadn't talked to Lynn in a couple of weeks, I asked about her. The husband of the couple said, "Lynn just got hired by Ford Motors to act in a commercial without an audition."

His wife asked, "How did they know she fit the part?"

He replied, "I guess it was from her promotional material. All I know is they phoned and that it's a pretty good bit of money for her."

Act the part and you'll get the job. Being healthy works the same way. Act healthful and you get to play that role too. Likewise, you pay the price, and nobody else, for acting sick. If the people you love are sick, then waste no time sitting around feeling bitter, lost, and forlorn.

I didn't make up this stuff myself. I'm not that smart. People have proven the power of words, thoughts, and emotions long before I was ever born.

To carry a burden violates spiritual law

"Every person has the power to bless and to multiply, to heal and to prosper. Words and thoughts have a tremendous vibratory force. What a person images, sooner or later, externalizes in their affairs. What they feel deeply or image clearly is impressed upon the subconscious mind, and carried out in minutest detail. Nothing stands between us and our highest ideals and every desire of the heart except doubt and fear."
Florence Scovel Shinn

My nineteen year-old son, Art, came to me about six months ago. He told me that he felt burdened because he did not know how he would attend college. I suggested that he imagine that he was already in college. How did it feel? What was his biggest joy as a college student?

After high school, Art had taken a year off to work and save money for college, but it wasn't going too well. He barely had a thousand dollars saved in the bank and didn't even have a car. On top of that he had failed Spanish his senior year of high school and so was unable to graduate. We decided he needed to take the GED test and then attend a community college and transfer to a four year school after making excellent grades. But Art felt discouraged and stuck in his work as a bus boy at a restaurant.

I encouraged him to begin feeling himself a success in school, to walk around the college campus and talk to the counselors there. He did this and a counselor helped him apply for grant money. While this was pending, he passed the GED test and spotted an old Volvo for sale along the road and had just enough cash to pay for it. Then he was accepted into community college and received grants in excess of his tuition, so he received a check from his college that allowed him to purchase a new lap top computer. Now Art is riding high.

The other day he said to me, "I want to learn all I can about the laws of creative visualization."

I replied, "No matter how much you learn about it, it always comes down to one thing -- surrender."

"What do you mean?" he asked.

"Never carry a burden," I explained. "Our job is simply to want good things and allow them to come to us as gifts."

As Art understands that truth and lives it, I've accomplished my job as a parent. And I would tell that same thing to anybody.

"Our job is simply to want good things."

Hold to your dreams

A client expressed that she felt immobilized. She said, "I always feel like I am stuck." Since she was well-versed in creative visualization, I asked her, "What if those words you just said were an affirmation? Would you wake up in the morning and say them?"

My clients as a group are spiritually attuned and seem to appreciate my banter on it. It has surprised me, however, how many people allow themselves to be in the dumps.

I often share a story Florence Scovel Shinn told in *The Game of Life*. She had a client, for whatever reason, who wanted a new set of dishware. The two of them agreed that she should receive that. Not long after, somebody gave Florence's client a single plate with a crack in it. She contacted Florence saying how typical that was of her, to want something and then get it with cracks.

Florence said -- no, do not stop at the cracked plate. Her client had merely magnetized the idea of receiving dishes and this cracked plate was a sign of things to come. When they held onto the original desire of receiving a beautiful set of new china dishes, it came.

For those who have "tried" creative visualization and found that it "didn't work," go back and ask yourself if you stopped believing after receiving "a cracked plate." This holds true for wanting healthy relationships, prosperity, anything. Get out of the dumps and continue looking for that which you have magnetized to draw into your world. Then plumb your thoughts and words in line with your desire.

A client said to me, "The bird flu is coming!"

I wondered to myself why anybody would ever want to magnetize that idea.

"Get out of the dumps and continue looking for that which you have magnetized to draw into your world."

Take no offense

Wayne Dyer said something on one of his CDs that is worth repeating. He pointed out that many people go through their day feeling offended by everything around them.

I confess, I'm guilty of that.

What offends me? Semi-trucks driving slowly in the passing lane on a freeway. A slow checker in a grocery store. Stupid headlines in the newspaper. Certain political bumper stickers. Dumb comments. Prejudice. Unfairness. Bigotry. Spite.

The list could go on. All day I can find circumstances to trigger my ire. If I review my life I can think of things I've done that would offend me now. Pretty weird, huh? I offend *myself*!

Back when I was a strict fundamentalist Christian, "the world" itself was offensive and I thought that it was my spiritual duty to foil crimes against me and Jesus. I consider myself fortunate to have outgrown that mode of chronic virulence.

Something that followed me wherever I went my whole life has been somebody else's incompetence tracking mud into my world. At any point during my career as an adult I could tell you (in great detail) all about somebody who was letting me down. In my mind then, if I could just be free of that person, everything would be grand. It took me years to see the pattern -- as soon as I ridded myself of one pain in my neck, another would knock on my door, usually offering me worse agony than the previous person.

"Taking offense" creates professional situations that are virtual torture. What happens in a structured job hierarchy is that you can obsess over certain personalities above you who might limit your rise to the top, and those who are below are almost certain to hinder you as well. From your own vantage, you then spend half your day beating up those in the organization who are not an adoring ally.

What happened with me was that I kept shrinking the organizations for which I worked until I could drown my professional enemies in a bath tub. Finally, I got my work down to two people, just me and one other, Chelsea, my business partner in colonics. Our initial attraction was that she hated her job as a nurse and I felt somewhat attracted to her hating her job as a nurse. It was an identification of sorts that together we needed to buck all hierarchy and live simply by our charm and our wits.

Chelsea and I spent every bit of savings we each had in the bank to open our office. Then we needed customers, which was my department, marketing. I sent mailings to previous massage customers and to a list of those in Nashville who already had gone for colonic treatments. I included both my phone number and Chelsea's because I needed her to succeed in order to continue paying her half of the bills.

Right away, Chelsea got calls, about five times as many as I received. Apparently, a female colon hygienist is preferred to a male. Thing was, this made Chelsea a hair too giddy. She asked me, "Are you jealous?" Wow, that made me mad. What bothered me was that I had done most of the work to establish the office and was now detecting an *attitude*. I decided the healthiest approach was to show her no hint as to how I really felt about her success -- success won all on my back.

Of course, *I* had no attitude.

Things started going wrong at the office. Chelsea's first offense: coming into the office, I found a huge turd floating in the toilet after her appointment. I immediately got her on the phone and chewed her out for this lack of attention to detail. The next time I went into the office the toilet was clean, but I found hair all over the bathroom floor, like somebody had been given a haircut. "Chelsea," I asked her over the phone, "Why is there hair all over the floor?"

"I'm so sorry!" she explained, "I cut my hair and forgot to sweep it up."

Another time I went into the office and found the massage table bearing a perfect body print in oil. Apparently she was giving a client a massage using my oil and didn't use a towel to cover the table.

The story behind that was that Chelsea and I had our own towels that we kept in a cabinet and she kept using *my* towels for her customers. When I complained that she needed to manage her own towels, she informed me that sometimes she needed to use my towels because she hadn't had time to wash hers. You get the picture. I solved my problem by keeping none of my towels in the room and brought fresh towels with me to each appointment. Now you understand why Chelsea had no towel for her client and why I was constantly simmering at a low boil.

Nothing I did was improving Chelsea. I tried phoning her after each offense and then I tried ignoring them. I created a list of chores needing to be done and we alternated weeks taking responsibility for completing various tasks. Once completed, chores were to be initialed, and the reason for this was so that I would have proof in black and white that she was not carrying her fair share of the load maintaining our office.

When I confronted her, she said that the office didn't need upkeep because it was always spotless when she went there and I replied, gnashing my teeth, "That's because *I* constantly clean it."

Finally, Chelsea began missing appointments with clients and they would call me because my business card was on the door. At least three times I rushed over to give Chelsea's client a colonic and because they had already paid Chelsea, I was never compensated.

At this point I had a heart-to-heart conversation with myself. It was obvious that Chelsea would not change after about a year and a half of bickering with her. There was only one thing remaining to do -- change *myself.* In a flash of epiphany, I accepted total responsibility for my propensity throughout my career to have an enemy at work. I released my stubborn need to always be right and the victim. I pictured Chelsea and sent her love -- not my love necessarily, but God's love, seeing her as perfect in every way.

A funny thing happened -- immediately. Chelsea stopped showing up at the office, period, the end. She didn't return my calls, nothing. After a couple of weeks, I phoned Chelsea's mother and she told me that Chelsea had vanished off the map.

Wow -- it felt a bit lonely. Took some getting used to. After about three weeks Chelsea phoned and explained that she had been taking some pretty hard drugs and had gotten herself into some bad situations and was calling me from a rehab center. She apologized profusely as she told me she wouldn't be back and that I could take possession of the office and her client list.

Wow, again!

"There was only one thing remaining to do -- change myself."

A couple of months later Chelsea phoned and asked if I could give her a ride somewhere. She wasn't looking too good. As she got out of the car she told me that she had lost everything -- her apartment, her mother had adopted her young daughter, she had no car. She had no money. She shrugged and said, "I am homeless now." I felt a rush of compassion watching her walk away from my car.

What I realized in her absence was that *without* Chelsea, I never would have been re-introduced to colonics. In many ways I owed her my life. For having blessed Chelsea, what returned to me was an overwhelming sense of gratitude.

She has since phoned me asking if she could come to the office to give herself a colonic, or her sister a colonic, or give her boyfriend a colonic, and I always welcome her. Chelsea and I became family. And after Chelsea uses the office these days, it always looks spotless.

Chelsea returned to work as a nurse and fell deeply in love with an amazing boyfriend who stuck by her side through many a tough time. They had a child together. The first time she came back to the office she drove an old beater car she had gotten at a junk yard for $300. Then she was driving a fairly decent older model SUV.

Now she looks like a typical mom, three years after being homeless, driving a mini-van.

There's more to the story. Our landlord had a discussion with Chelsea when she was at the peak of her troubles and he offered to give her a two-month reprieve on her share of the rent. It ended up extending to six months until he had me sign a new lease. We had been paying him one hundred dollars over the initial rent charge and when the lease came in for me to sign, the rent was lowered by $150.

It was like the maximum happy ending and it taught me a wonderful lesson. Avoid taking offense. Bless your enemies. Better yet, have no enemies.

That is the part of Christianity that works. Jesus came not to condemn the world, but to love it. I'm thinking I'll stick with that aspect of spirituality, and when you get down to it, being right all the time does stink.

Surrendering the need to be right releases the angels of our better nature. And you wouldn't want to trip up those little babies.

Chapter Nine
Clean the colon -- final answer

"No animal in nature ever eats such a haphazard comminglement of heterogeneity."

Herbert M. Shelton, *Food Combining Made Easy*

By now you could be thinking, "Isn't Mr. Webb finished yet?" Man, I'm cranking as fast as I can. You can now better imagine how difficult it is for me to reply to clients who ask, "Tell me about colon hygiene." I have files of articles I have collected over the years that I haven't even tapped into.

Someone phoned yesterday and told me how reading Dr. Norman Walker's books about diet and internal cleansing changed her life. I've never read his books, knowing that I should. A few years ago a client brought in a book written by Dr. Richard Anderson. He's written wonderful stuff about internal cleansing with full color photos and I haven't taken the time to read him either. These are also untapped reservoirs.

One author I have read is Jay Kordich, also known as "Jay the Juiceman." He introduced me to the raw powers of fresh fruits and vegetables. I believe he knew Dr. Norman Walker personally.

I have not read *all* of what Jordan S. Rubin, N.M.D. has written, maybe half. And I've flipped through much of what Brenda Watson, N.D. and Leonard Smith, M.D. have written and I applaud their thorough investigations. Of course, Dr. Bernard Jensen is an ultimate authority on diet and cleansing the gut. He wrote at least ten books, probably way more, but I've only read two. But I've read those two at least three times.

I doubt I'll write another book on the topic of internal cleansing. By the time I have caught up on all I haven't read, you will have already beat me to it. Then you'll be the expert on cleaning the colon.

Seriously, you take it from here. My story is mostly completed.

Some old school stuff will always be classic. Like Herbert M. Shelton. How could a person express it better than to tell it like he does in the above quote? "Haphazard comminglement of heterogeneity" -- that's classically pure poetry if I ever heard it. Some things just can't be improved.

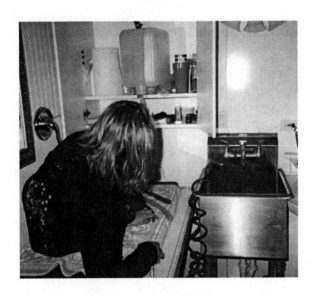

Susan's home unit installed in her basement.

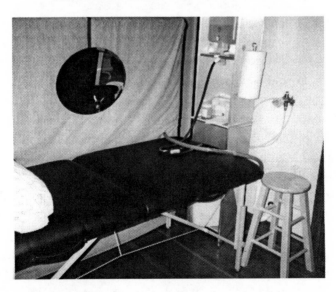

Gravity-flow colonic unit with five gallon tank and hoses.

Types of poop

I have now told you most of what I know about poop and health. Being healthy today comes down to cleaning the colon. That is my final answer.

What comes out of the body from a bowel movement on the toilet compared to what exits during a colonic are two very different animals. Usually poop in the toilet is some shade of brown and appears like smooth clay. What shakes loose from the colon during a colonic can be five to ten times longer and includes mucus, usually not seen in the toilet. Often it comes through the colonic tube wrapped like bacon around the feces.

Sometimes pure mucus comes out in a variety of colors ranging from tan to bright white. It can appear leafy, like seaweed, or I've seen it perfectly braided in lengths 12 to 18 inches long. If it is leafy, it is translucent; if braided or in ropes, opaque. I believe that mucus can stick to the colon wall and grow in length like stalactites on the roof of a cave. There might be times when poop comes through the colon in a corkscrew fashion which twists mucus rope into braids. Otherwise I don't know how it's braided.

"What comes out of the body from a bowel movement on the toilet compared to what exits during a colonic are two very different animals."

This mucus must be tough because it appears like rope. The more colonics a person does, the more of this mucus stuff you see. Most colonic sessions also release small flakes of mucus, like potato flakes. At the end of the colonic, you might see about two cups of these flakes exit in the water.

Initial colonics produce the basic poop you see in the toilet. Colonics increase the volume dramatically and it makes absolutely no difference whether the person has just had a bowel movement or even done an enema. The average release during a colonic is three to five feet long.

It makes little difference whether a person is fat or thin as to the volume of poop which might exit. Thin people actually seem to release more.

The personality of the colon is that of a trickster. It fools me all the time. Sometimes I might tell a client that "they are done" and immediately a rush of fecal matter floods out. Colon hygiene stays fascinating because you never know what to expect.

People going through transitional periods, like a divorce or a career change, seem to release more. Emotions seem to stimulate action. I have often told people that psychiatrist couches need little colonics units installed because crying, laughing, and anger releases deeply held volumes of fecal matter. Any subject of emotional importance seems to pry stuff loose from the colon like shaking apples from a tree.

The longer the colonic's duration, the more productive the colonic. Generally a person will have a major release of fecal matter with moderate cramping after about twenty minutes. If you wait another twenty minutes, a second rush releases. The second rush involves more intense cramping and includes about a quart of filthy water ranging from bright yellow to orange to chocolate in color.

After the colonic finishes, a person usually feels the need to have a bowel movement on the toilet. This releases anything from clean-appearing water, to filthy water, to more fecal matter, and sometimes just gas. Generally the odor of anything removed after the colonic is putrid and foul. The only person I am aware of who has released a substantial amount of toxic ammonia after a colonic, is me.

The pain experienced during a colonic ranges from none to extreme. One woman grabbed my arm and squeezed it hard as tears burst from her eyes uncontrollably. Some people flinch, others moan -- sometimes loudly! Cramping is a sign of a cooperative bowel.

Lots of people ask about gas. Here's the fallacy: people picture gas in their gut like it's bubbles in a garden hose. They forget about ballooning of fecal matter in the colon and don't think about constrictions. They don't imagine muscle tone being lost in the colon. Under those conditions, gas gets trapped and painful. Chronic bloating can be a serious issue. I've found that the clients who are very ill have the most gas volume.

Stinky farts and bloating are not the same. I've done lots of internal cleansing and I still get gas. Just ask my kids. But I rarely get bloating. Bloating means cleansing the colon with water is a good idea. Bloated clients get fast relief from colonics.

Clients sometimes ask me during a colonic, "Is that old stuff?" My opinion is that "old stuff" won't release until at least twenty colonics.

This past summer, one client did fifty colonics. She began doing three per week and when she reached twenty five, we saw black fecal matter like charcoal exit. That's the old stuff. The first time the length was about four feet. I told her she was in a transformational state and needed to return the next day. Another four feet of black stuff came out. She returned the next day, same result. Nine days in a row, this happened and then the charcoal-stuff stopped. Keep in mind that this client was eating no solid food because she was on a 90-day juice fast.

Fasting is a great idea for concentrated cleansing along with colonics. An enema removes fecal matter from the sigmoid area, but probably not much deeper. It makes me nervous to think of people running enema tubing high into the colon. This fall I gave colonics to a group participating in a week-long juice fast and some did this form of enema, but then the colonic *still* removed ungodly amounts of additional fecal matter.

If an enema bag is all you have, do an enema. The question of whether enemas make a person dependent on them is answered when you see what comes out.

"Fasting is a great idea for concentrated cleansing along with colonics."

Author Edgar Cayce published a map of the colon showing that it has reflex points. Reflex points represent energetic or nerve correlations connected to other points and organs in the body. The human body has many places commonly accepted as reflexive -- the eyes, ears, feet and hands, to name a few. Cayce stated that by filling the colon with water, it stimulates a healing response throughout the entire body.

Another interesting fact: when the human body is formed in the womb, the brain and the gut divide from the same neural network. Early on, the fetus is mostly a head with a gut and the body develops out of the gut. The gut connects to everything.

Since I am also a massage therapist, I have observed that my clients who get a colonic feel relaxed from warm water being put into the gut as if their whole body received a massage. I've had clients report neck pain disappear after a colonic and that their legs feel lighter. That corroborates Edgar Cayce's findings.

And a colonic can often alleviate a bad headache.

Sometimes I witness a length of fecal matter longer than the colon itself -- seven or eight feet of poop from a five-foot long colon. I believe this additional stuff comes from an impacted or "stuffed" section of the colon.

When I worked as a massage therapist for a chiropractor, the doctor showed me an X-ray outline of a patient's sigmoid area near the rectum and it appeared to be stretched-out like it held three large grapefruits. The doctor said this ballooning of the colon was **common** to see on an X-ray.

The pelvis is shaped like a bowl. There is no reason to dispute that this bowl can fill to overflowing. The colon does have the ability to stretch and swell. A healthy colon would be about two inches in diameter while an unhealthy colon could be nine inches across.

Vegetarian Times magazine (March, 1998), wrote: "As the old expression goes, death begins in the colon. Don't believe it? Ask any coroner. Autopsies often reveal colons that are plugged up to 80 percent with waste material."

A colon stuffed full might have a passage way the size of a pencil. If the colon itself is constricted or pinched, the opening could be just as small. If a bowel movement in the toilet appears thin or ribbon-like, that indicates ballooning or a constriction. If you have this type of poop, do not panic. It is just a call to pay attention to your diet in relation to the shape and dimension of your poop. If you eat more fresh, organic fruit, vegetables, and salads, observe improvements in your bowel habits and dimensions.

Fast food burgers and fries always produces fecal matter like concrete. Seriously -- how can it not?

People who eat plant matter and do not chew, will have a colonic which reveals their lack of chewing. I have seen whole lettuce and spinach leaves come out perfectly intact during a colonic. Nuts and mushrooms are notorious for slipping past the teeth. Once I saw twenty almonds come through the tubing without a single bite mark and the client acknowledged eating them in a hurry. I mean, a big hurry!

"With humans, chewing is vital to the digestive process."

When I was a kid, I watched my dog eat and modeled my own chewing behavior after that of a canine -- three chews and a swallow. However, animals designed to eat other animals have shorter digestive tracts and about twenty times the stomach acid intensity to digest skin, and fur, and to kill bacteria on a rancid carcass.

With humans, chewing is vital to the digestive process. Coating food in saliva facilitates better digestion. Plant matter cannot be broken down by the type of human enzymes produced and therefore only what is *chewed* can be assimilated. That is why juicing fresh vegetables brings maximum benefit because the cellulose material is broken apart so the body can access the nutritional value.

Some fruits like pineapple, no matter how much it is chewed, still comes through the colonic tubing looking like pineapple. Believe it or not, so does watermelon, unless it's totally pulverized in the mouth. I've seen watermelon exit during my colonic thirty minutes after eating it. So, moving from mouth to anus can be as fast as thirty minutes or as long as twenty or thirty years. Generally I see what has been eaten within 24 hours. After twenty colonics, old layers start to exfoliate.

Does watermelon passing within 30 minutes mean that the digestive tract is otherwise perfectly clean of other fecal matter?

Not in the slightest! It slides past old fecal matter that has become stuck in mucus along the colon wall.

When people tell me that they eat a healthy diet, I ask them how they ate ten or twenty years earlier. The colon's health is cumulative in nature.

Many people have small pebble-like rabbit turds plop into the toilet. This is not from eating "rabbit food," but from eating rabbit. Those rocks are made from animal protein and white flour. Sometimes the pebbles will stick together like a nut-bar. Basically, that is an indicator to eat more salad and natural plant fiber -- rabbit *food*.

When fecal matter releases into the colonic tubing, it either floats or sinks. Floating stuff indicates more fiber content, while low-flying poop indicates heavy protein content. You want to remove heavy proteins from the colon. *Bacillus coli* is a mean-spirited bacteria that eats poorly digested proteins in the gut and then poisons the entire body. High meat intake surely leads to dark, puffy circles under the eyes.

Clients ask me about parasites. When I was a kid, we caught our own worms for fishing. We snuck up on them at night with flashlights and grabbed them before they could slide back down into their holes. A big night crawler will put up a fight and if you ever battle one you will discover that worms are strong and they are smart.

National Geographic made a bold statement about parasites in a documentary titled, "The Body Snatchers." This film stated: "Parasites have killed more humans than all the wars in history."

If you are a person with a ballooned section in your colon, filled with old rotting fecal matter, forget fighting worms. They can quickly slide into a ready-made bunker you helped build. I think most of the herbal parasite cleansing systems on the market are a joke. But if you find one that works, by all means, have at it. Understand that what you can see exit into the toilet represents a fraction of your infestation.

The best defense against human parasites is to clean house -- their house! Flooding the colon with water can break apart their homes and pull out weaker and younger worms. I don't see them during a colonic because worms don't generally come out alive. If they die, they deteriorate quickly inside the body.

Sometimes poop leaves the body fizzing. It looks like it has one of those bubbling tablets stuck on it -- *that much* fizz! What that means -- the poop is fermenting to such a degree that it exits as if from a champagne bottle. Fizz indicates yeast in the gut. You want that stuff out because larger parasites like to live in fizz. I've also seen the colonic tubing totally fill with foam like you might see shooting from a beer can.

I suggest people forget worms and just cleanse the colon. And supplement good bacteria. In my opinion, the worst parasites are not the big ones, but the zillions of single-cell bacteria and yeast fungus. They are like tiny bees creating poisonous honey inside the gut. Call it pus. Bigger parasites love eating it like a delicacy.

When my kids were younger, they both had pin worms and lice. I'm not sure which was worse. They took pin worm medicine. Since I've gone natural, we haven't had pin worms, so I don't know how to treat them naturally. Search the Internet for that.

I suspect that I have more internal yeast fungus than I should have, however, I still have mercury fillings in my teeth and I've read that yeast can act to counter mercury in the body. This is one of the beautiful aspects of colon cleansing. It takes the strategy out of getting well. You cleanse the body of toxic stuff and don't worry about treating parasites like worms or Candida yeast.

When you start "self-medicating," you can affect balances in the body that your logic and mind get totally wrong. You might go crazy to clear yourself of yeast and then lose the form of protection it provided the body against heavy metals.

I question taking handfuls of supplements because I believe the best medicine comes in healthy organic raw fruits and vegetables. Scientists admit that there is still much, much more to learn about health and diet. My bet is that the fuzz on a peach has healing properties yet to be discovered, as does the strings in celery, etc., etc.

Clean the gut, eat smart, and don't think so much.

I just helped a client install a colonics unit in her home. The plumber told her that he knew a friend who had done a colonic, but it sent her to the emergency room because "it severed an internal polyp." My client was fairly distraught.

I suggested to my client to ask more questions the next time somebody disparaged colonics. "Who had the polyp? How old were they? Can I get their phone number? Are you sure it was from *colonics* and not from a colonoscopy?" I have never once found that a colonic injured anybody and the more questions I ask, the more revealing the story.

I had a literary agent interested in representing me, but then she wrote me an email stating that she wouldn't pursue it because she heard the latest information -- "colonics are damaging to health." I wrote her asking for more details and didn't hear back. I sent her a second email stating that we were in a professional discussion and it was irresponsible of her to make a negative claim about my topic without documentation.

She sent a reply. She said that she couldn't *exactly recall*, but that her information came from a television talk show. I replied with two words: "It figures."

I have seen blood only one time during a colonic and that was from a client with cancer. I noticed the water turn pink and then more pink. I asked, "Have you been eating beets?" The reply was, "No." The pink color faded within ten seconds and it stopped. But out of thousands of colonics, that was the only fresh blood I've seen. If blood inside the colon was old, it would be dark, and I've not seen this either.

I have seen undissolved pills come out of people, but rarely. One client took about twenty potassium tablets per day and generally we saw twenty tablets come through the tubing. When she switched to capsules, that stopped. My mother did a colonic and when I set the speculum in the sink a green pill fell out still fizzing. Some people ask whether I see lots of pills or childhood toys or gum and the answer is no.

The other common question I get is why camera pictures of the colon during a colonoscopy show a pink, healthy organ? That's a good one. I've never seen a film of a colonoscopy and I'd love to. I think colon hygienists should be a part of the process.

The questions I have is: "If the colonoscopy process cleans the colon, why do Americans suffer from colon ballooning in record numbers? Couldn't doctors cleanse the colon in one-fell swoop?

Why do X-rays show a ballooned colon that doesn't change after the colonoscopy? Why are the colons of cadavers generally ballooned?"

I've given colonics to people following a colonoscopy and seen not only fecal matter exit, but about a gallon of chalky water come out. I think gastroenterologists should sit through some colonic sessions and explain what the hell is going on. I've written a letter to a local gastroenterologist whom I heard was progressive and never got a reply.

"If the colonoscopy process cleans the colon, why do Americans suffer from colon ballooning in record numbers?"

Truth is, there's a lot yet to discover. Mystery can be enthralling. But I wouldn't wait till all the answers are in before starting to clean your colon by flushing it with water. Poop might just become the latest frontier.

Your frontier. Because you and I know you have plenty of poop inside.

What to eat

"Man is trying to teach Nature how to grow and that will never do."
Alan Chadwick, *Villa Montalvo Lecture Series*

Clients frequently ask me what I recommend for diet. Sometimes, when I tell them they should eat whatever they want, they get frustrated. They'll ask me what *I* eat.

Okay -- here's what I eat. My diet has slowly evolved into this because I have less time today than I used to have to give myself colonics. I eat mainly to feel light like I could fly off and run at a moment's notice. If I eat until I feel sluggish and full, then eventually it works its way down to my colon and then it feels full and gross. Then I feel forced to give myself a colonic.

For that reason, I am converting to a mostly raw diet of fresh, organic fruits and vegetables, seeds, and nuts. My goal is to be converted by this time next year, maybe sooner. By then I will have eliminated meat and dairy and packaged products, I think.

For breakfast I usually eat fruit. This summer I ate watermelon almost daily. Now pears are in season and on sale, so I ate pears this morning and brought fresh pears to my two kids for breakfast.

Since it was beautiful outside, I paid my daughter $6 for her time to go jogging with me at the track. My son joined us, but I didn't pay him because he has plenty of money. The main objective was to get sun and breathe fresh air.

The past couple days I've splurged buying wild Alaskan salmon, mainly because it's been incredibly delicious. I drizzle it with a grape seed oil, pure maple syrup, some Celtic sea salt, and cayenne pepper and then broil it.

Along with the fish I made a huge salad of organic baby arugula leaves, which I bought for half price on sale. I sprinkled a fresh salad dressing on it and some probiotic powder. I also made some nutra-farmed brown rice which I cooked in filtered water, sea salt, and while it cooled I added olive oil to it.

Oh -- thirty minutes before eating the fish I fed my kids each about 3 tablespoons of Udo's Choice essential oil on a spoon with an orange juice chaser, organic, purchased on sale. Sometimes we take Garden of Life coconut oil instead -- change things up. And we take Garden of Life's *Primal Defense* probiotic, but I change that up too, and switch to another brand every other time.

We used to drink soy milk, but I switched to almond milk because there's questionable things about soy. Lots of opinions going around, but not life and death.

A few hours after feeding my daughter I noticed that she had picked at her food. I asked her about it and she said she didn't like it. Next thing I knew she was in the kitchen looking into the freezer. She found a package of "Putney Pasta" -- Butternut Squash and Vermont Maple Syrup Ravioli and said that is what she wanted.

It took me five minutes to prepare. I opened a can of organic tomatoes which I had bought when it was on sale for a dollar. I chopped two cloves of fresh garlic, some onion, and spinach, adding it to the hot water as the ravioli softened. She tasted it saying it needed cheese, so I added about a dollar's worth of goat cheese to the finished mix which she devoured and praised.

Tonight I will eat fresh guacamole I made yesterday with organic blue corn chips. My son is in the kitchen right now with a friend eating Basha-brand hommus with chips.

Fairly standard to my diet is to eat a sprouted bread baked at low heat called Manna bread. It comes in a variety of grains and flavors. I eat it with raw almond butter. I also like to eat celery or apples with raw almond butter.

"When I first heard the theories behind the raw food diet, I knew immediately it was the way to go."

I have two raw food cookbooks and about twice a week I'll break out a recipe and try it. My last invention was a cauliflower salad made from tahini sauce and fresh garlic. I also made a fresh hommus, but it turned out a bit strong on the garlic. I ate it like medicine. The cauliflower salad gave me gas.

In my former diet I rarely ate fresh produce. Back then I got my spinach from packaged foods that had spinach as one of the ingredients. I rarely ate real pears or apples or salads.

When I first heard the theories behind the raw food diet, I knew immediately it was the way to go. Eating cooked food might have worked before farming became so toxic, but now raw organic fruits and vegetables are required as cleansing tools to undo the damages. Once you discover the produce department, it can be thrilling. In many countries it is not possible to eat only raw food because it is not available year around like it is in America.

I eat a salad almost every day. There are so many types of salad ingredients I never get tired of eating it. The main point is to chew it well because it won't digest if it isn't chewed. Pine nuts on any salad makes it exquisite.

I would never eat a salad from a fast food restaurant. Here's why -- read this excerpt from the May, 2005 issue of *Ode* magazine: **The**

underside of salad. "Pre-washed lettuce sold in plastic bags and ready for the salad bowl is one of the latest success stories for the ready-made food industry. But it comes at a price. The catalogue of the hip British sustainable clothing manufacturer **Howies** (autumn/ winter 2004/2005) offered the recipe for washed salad:

Firstly, add four pinches of insecticides. Two pinches of fungicide. And two measures of herbicide. After picking, store in conditions that reduce the oxygen from 21% to 3% and replace with the corresponding amount of CO_2. This is perfect now for stopping the aging process so the salad still appears fresh, but it can't stop the goodness from being lost with each day that passes. Keep in this state for anything up to a month. Then take some chlorine, 50 mg per litre should do it (a measure the equivalent of 20 times the strength of your local swimming pool) and gently rinse. Then simply bag. Ready for sale. Supermarkets. Now wash your hands of that."

I would say: Fast Food. Equally toxic methods. Wash your hands of that.

Lots of clients tell me that they can't afford to eat organic food. I can buy organic salad fresh at the salad bar for $5.99 per pound. A half-pound salad costs $3. A quarter pound hamburger and fries weighs roughly the same, a half-pound. What's the cost diff?

Organic apples right now are on sale for 99 cents per pound. You can eat apples all day for that. And organic spinach is 99 cents per bunch on sale.

I used to figure in my mind how pesticides were sprayed and tried to scrimp on food that grew under the ground, like regular potatoes sometimes are five pounds for a dollar. But then I read somewhere that food grown under the ground gets saturated in chemicals. Then I read that strawberries have the worst pesticide and preservative residue. So I quit trying to second guess farming methods and now only eat organic.

It used to be that if I ate a strawberry, it had been squished into a frosted Pop Tart -- maybe one berry per box. It's a whole new experience to shop the produce section. I've discovered that produce grows in seasons. Imagine that!

My grandfather always grew a garden, even well into his eighties, and I have never grown a garden. I mistakenly did not eat his produce because it looked dirty and imperfect. I know better now. So that will be one of my great joys some day -- to grow a garden.

The past couple summers I have been invited to raid other people's gardens. What a treat that has been -- to pick a tomato and pop it directly into my mouth. To see the bugs and spiders crawling around the food. To pick a cucumber and discover it has rough hairs growing on it in the wild garden. I tell you I've become a real country boy!

I don't cook in aluminum. Haven't used a microwave in years. I avoid eggs that come from factory farms. It's worth an extra ten cents per egg to get them organic. Research "factory farming" on the Internet and you'll see why. Read some of the articles online at www.acresUSA.com.

I would like to juice vegetables every day, but it's usually once a week. But I will have good stretches where I juice daily.

If I buy bottled juice, it's been pasteurized, which means the life has been cooked out of it. What I'll do is use it as a "carrier medium" for my kids to supplement greens or sea vegetables or flax oil. We don't drink soft drinks much. I buy bottled water instead and keep a steady supply.

If we eat in a restaurant, we eat whatever we want. There is almost no way that food making its way into a restaurant will be grown in a healthy way, so give it up. Just eat it. I might eat at a Subway, but prefer not to. The vegetables usually look limp and pale.

This summer we were on the road and I saw a sign for a fast food chicken restaurant we used to love that had the best Cajun red beans and rice. I decided to pull off the freeway to get the red beans, but once there, I yielded to ordering some spicy chicken too. While we waited, my daughter pointed to the back counter at giant blocks of white lard and asked, "What's that?"

I replied, "That's what they're cooking our chicken in."

The lobby stunk like disinfectant, but the floor had permanent stains everywhere. The woman at the front counter turned and yelled to the back of the kitchen, "Where's Harold? We need biscuits." Somebody shouted back, "He's changing the grease." The experience was reminding me why I was switching to raw foods.

So then we finally get back to the car and my daughter says, "I didn't get a biscuit." I went back inside and cut to the front of the line and got a biscuit. When I opened my box, I found no red beans, just fries, which I didn't order. So I trudged back inside again and by now the lady at the counter was sweating so badly that it was literally dripping off her nose. I felt determined to get my red beans and watched the ball of sweat hanging to make sure my food wasn't splashed with a sweaty drop.

I'm sorry to say that I ate two bites of my chicken and had to throw it out. It tasted like it had soap on it. I told my kids that if you imagined the mistakes we didn't know about as our food came to market -- knowing the mistakes we *did* see during the ten minutes we were there -- the food was most likely not edible.

It's not like I've become a snob. I've eaten pork rinds from a bag like anybody else. It's just that I no longer *want* processed food when I can eat fresh stuff. I mean, eating a big old slice of cool watermelon makes me feel happy.

For those eating the low carb, high protein diet, God help you. You are going to be as constipated as a rock. If you're stuck on it, understand that green leafy salad acts like a digestive shock absorber between mouthfuls of meat.

An interesting advantage with the raw food diet is the fact that the human body is mostly water. As we age, we dehydrate. We get wrinkled. Babies don't get wrinkles because they are about 90 percent liquid. Old people are more dry.

Raw fruits and vegetables are mostly water. I figure that it keeps you younger eating food that has high water content. When processed food is left out, it gets hard. Figure that's what happens in the body too. If cheese hardens as it ages, it will harden also inside your body and dry you up. When raw food goes bad it sags and melts. A rotten tomato is still wet.

I received an unsolicited email today warning folks against eating processed foods that have "MSG" as an ingredient. The author was very upset that fast food restaurants were using it to make their products more addictive. And many foods on the grocer's shelves contain MSG. The thing is, when you eat a raw organic tomato, you can relax knowing it will never contain MSG. The more raw organic produce you consume, the less chance you'll have for ingesting MSG.

When it gets down to it, eating raw organic produce simplifies a lot of questions about diet. The rule of thumb is: the less processed, the better.

Finally, this may sound difficult, but it's really not. In a social order driven by consumer choice, recognize that every time you spend a dollar on some product, you cast it like a vote of support. If you purchase food that has the Kraft label, then you have cast a vote of confidence that Kraft is supporting your best interests. Maybe so. Maybe not. If you take medicine from a particular pharmaceutical corporation, then that means you trust that corporation to make pills in your best interest to take.

"When it gets down to it, eating raw organic produce simplifies a lot of questions about diet."

What if they're not supporting your best interests while you support them?

The most important aspect to consider about diet is the nature of the corporations making the products which you willingly put into your body. Like, what do you know about the fast food corporations who want to sell you a salad? Or what do you know about the Dole corporation, which also wants to sell you a salad?

Many corporations rely on our blind trust that they make foods healthy to consume. Most folks will invest time researching television or computer brands before making a purchase and yet never think twice about who is making their dinner. And we might get paranoid about second-hand cigarette smoke and never notice power lines running next to the upstairs bedroom nor care about toxic chemicals in the hot tub.

The time has come to consider what's being done *to our land*. Adolf Hitler's primary admiration of America was how the government stole the land from the Indians. In his mind he was doing the same thing -- taking land from less-advanced peoples.

This theft continues to this day, except that it is pure technology that has been on the march.

Read the monthly newspaper, *Acres USA*, to learn more. Writer Joel Salatin will give it to you straight.

Those are my initial thoughts about diet. If I shared them with my clients there would be no time for the colonic. That is another reason why I encourage my clients to eat whatever they want. That way everybody is doing their own homework. But deep down, I'm quietly hoping people will start paying more attention to who makes their food (and medicines). Like discovering who's behind the box? Or just skipping the box.

One idea I have for the future is a new kind of progressive summer dinner party. Everybody dresses up in their finest and visits each other's gardens during the peak harvest and eats straight from the plants. Open a bottle of wine and that's the best concept I have for a person's ideal diet.

That's food locally grown, organic, ripe in season, eaten in loving community. The wine of course is optional, but I myself would not turn it down.

On my soap box

I watched a Public TV documentary about a guy who is a mobile butcher. He drives to farms and slaughters animals on site. His truck has a back unit like a large ambulance except all the equipment is for butchering.

He cleans the unit with a hose and lots of soap. If the customer has an animal raised on organic feed, the butcher uses iodine to clean surfaces instead of soap. That struck me as interesting.

I never had considered that non-organic meat might have soap residue on it. That would be an added chemical in addition to feed that probably had animal protein in it, antibiotics, hormones, and other man-made additives. It might not be much soap, but it's enough that they don't use any soap to clean if butchering an organic animal.

"I never had considered that non-organic meat might have soap residue on it."

It would stand to reason that the more a meat product is processed, the more surfaces it would pass over (and through) which were cleaned with soap. The meat that went into a hot dog, for example, would have more soap on it than a simple steak. And it has been demonstrated that the more processed a meat is, the more it causes cancer.

Here's what Nashville's local daily newspaper had to say:

"Take me out to the ball park ...
But cut way back on the hot dogs. A new study conducted by the World Health Organization finds that eating *preserved* meats such as salami, bacon, ham, and hot dogs can increase the risk of bowel cancer by fifty-percent. Previous studies linked high meat intake to colorectal cancer, but these studies grouped fresh and processed meats together. However, when it comes to fresh red meat -- beef, lamb, pork, and veal, there seems to be no link."
Source: *The Tennessean*

Now I'm wondering what studies have been done on the soap used to clean the equipment making preserved meats. Then I'm thinking about some kid eating a hot dog on vacation with sun screen and bug repellent on his skin, and taking some kind of pharmaceutical prescription chemical, munching on chips, washing it down with a soda. Then he's getting added sterilizer-soap on top of all that toxic input.

What the hell are we doing to him?

I'll get off my soap box now.

Parenting teens

My seventeen year old daughter started getting her menstrual cycle every two weeks. This continued for two months and she asked to see a doctor.

So, Maddie went to the doctor.

The doctor said that she needed to get onto birth control pills and that her menstrual cycle should return to normal within six months. Maddie asked the doctor for another option that might be more natural.

The doctor replied, "You are just being difficult."

So Maddie came home none the better. In the meantime, I started asking my clients about it. One client said she had the exact same problem and she has been taking birth control pills since and she suggested "not to do it."

"Why?" I asked surprised, since it helped.

"I hate taking the pills every single day," she said.

Another client was a nurse and she told me she took a contraceptive shot every six months and after two years happened to read the literature on it and noticed it said to check bone density after taking it for ... *two years*. She asked her O.B. about it and tests were made and the results came back that she was in an early stage of osteoporosis. Her bone loss was significant enough that she was taken off the contraceptive. At age 32.

"Did you ask your doctor for the test or did your doctor suggest that you take the test?" I asked.

"I asked for the test."

"Would your doctor have given you the test if you hadn't asked?"

"Her bone loss was significant enough that she was taken off the contraceptive."

"I'm pretty sure," she replied, "Yes." Then she added, "I filled out a questionnaire and one of the questions was whether I drank diet soda and I *was* drinking diet soda, so I quit drinking it then and there. If they correlated it to bone loss, I was over it."

My informal quizzing was not leaning me towards putting Maddie onto birth control pills. Instead, I started personally giving her the *Udo's Choice* oil on a spoon right into her mouth. Before that I just assumed she was taking it because it was in the refrigerator. I started juicing more vegetables. And I took her to the track to jog and get some sunshine. We also went shopping together for some new clothes.

I realized that I had been assuming that we spent enough time together since we lived in the same house. When I really looked at it, I wasn't spending near enough time with my beautiful seventeen year-old daughter. Whatever it was, her period returned to normal. We'll continue to monitor it, but my conclusion is that Maddie needed more father attention.

And that's the thing. If you're the father of a teen girl and you don't pay attention, somebody in a professional capacity might be telling your precious child to take toxic little pills. And they might be bullying her, too, saying stuff like, "You're being difficult."

And that's just not true. Dads should stand up to that crap.

More on a better diet

My client, Chen, came to see me today. I asked him about his diet lately.

"I've been eating chicken and macaroni and cheese," he said, "Black people food."

I asked him, "What's 'black people food'?"

"You know, fried food ..."

"What about salads?" I asked.

"No," he said smiling, "Salad's not black people food."

"Well," I said, "Then salad's got to become black people food."

He replied, "In my part of town, you can't get good salad."

"I understand," I said, "And that's got to change too."

Evidence that demands a verdict

Chen's friend, Gwen, had an appointment after him. Nothing came out of her colon after two tanks of water and I said to her, "Your poop is hard inside."

She replied, "I'm not constipated. I go every day."

"Just because you go doesn't mean you're not constipated," I said.

"How do you know?" she asked.

"That is a really good question," I said. I explained to her what I knew.

A medical study was done in England that took years to complete. I don't know who sponsored it, but researchers asked people whether they were constipated. I believe the number of participants was 500 and only about twelve said they were chronically backed-up. After each of the 500 died, the colon was analyzed. The colons of 488 had significant congestion. Exactly the opposite of what people had thought.

That correlates with my findings as a colonic therapist. Ninety-eight percent of the colons I fill with water show signs of constipation.

"If I'm constipated," Gwen asked, "Why don't I know it?"

I placed my finger on her arm. "Do you feel that?" I asked her. "Yes."

"If I kept my finger on you, eventually you wouldn't feel it," I explained. "Constipation begins as a slight pressure and most people can't feel it. I know I couldn't feel it either and I was horribly constipated -- stuffed full."

We think of our digestive tract like it's a garden hose. It's much more lumpy and bumpy than that. It's designed for surface area, not as a slippery slide. It is designed more for uptake than output.

Imagine driving to a remote forest and being thrown out and told to survive on what you can find growing and living there. That's basically the history of the human diet. Imagine surviving through the winter months and you can understand why the digestive tract needed to squeeze every bit of energy from food.

The more surfaces inside the human body that a nut or berry

bumps against, the greater the likelihood it will be sucked up and burned as fuel. If a piece of chalk symbolized nutrition, then to get full advantage, it would be smarter to scratch chalk across a tennis court than to drop it into a garden hose. That's our surface area inside -- a tennis court. Fold it up into a gut and realize that we are mostly hollow in the middle.

Just appreciate that hollow is not the same as smooth.

"That's our surface area inside -- a tennis court."

Teeth are added to the equation, but what for? Imagine bouncing an apple across a tennis court. That represents a small surface area meeting a large surface area. If the apple is pulverized into apple sauce and spread thinly over the tennis court, the apple can cover a much, much broader surface area. If the goal is to suck the apple through the surface of the tennis court, then teeth represent the stroke of genius in our design.

If you lived in the woods by an apple tree and that was your sole source of food, then eleven months of the year you would be hungry. During that time you would eat whatever you could find -- nuts, berries, leaves. Here and there a squirrel or a frog. The human system of the gut with teeth at the top has served the situation perfectly.

Now -- in your imagination -- stack a year's worth of food found in the woods into a large barrel. It's full of nuts, berries, leaves, some apples. Contrast that with a barrel filled with fast food meals. Sausage, eggs, bread, meat, fries, Coke. There's just no comparison. Especially not after pouring a pound of chemicals like turpentine over the barrel filled with fast food.

There have been many trade-offs as humans have progressed. One of those significant trade-offs is constipation.

There is more evidence that constipation has become widespread amongst civilized peoples. Diverticular diseases of the colon tell us a lot. In places on the planet where people still consume nuts, berries, leaves, and an occasional frog, nobody gets diverticular diseases.

My son, Art, discovered that the waitresses at the restaurant where he worked frequently talked about health and beauty amongst themselves and he started joining in the conversations. One day he pointed out that "before and after" pictures of women who had converted to the raw food diet showed dramatic improvements in appearance. One waitress said, "If I had the choice between aging badly or eating the raw food diet, I'd choose aging badly."

That's the thing. It's a choice. That's the best part. Making choices.

The trade-offs to eating the typical American diet are the unique American illnesses, dysfunctions, and pills. There is almost no gap between the health of those at the top of the food chain and those at the bottom. The menu at the golf course's cafe differs from fast food only that "ham" at the one means sandwich, while at the other it means burger.

"The trade-offs to eating the typical American diet are the unique American illnesses, dysfunctions, and pills."

If you want to see a gap, investigate the subculture of Americans eating raw nuts, fruits, leaves, and vegetables -- the organic culture. Or go back in time. Rent some old movies and notice how healthy those folks looked. What does it mean? Post World War II, civilized cultures have become increasingly constipated. We're living in the era of the full gut.

What's at stake? Has lifestyle come down to an "either-or"? To be or not to be -- constipated. Is that the question?

My friend, Susan, is a nurse, very smart. I bumped into her in the nutrition section of our local Wild Oats store talking to a clerk, whom I also knew. Susan was asking about natural means to treat her case of eczema that was no longer responding to medicines. She hiked her skirt to show her thighs. Each leg had about a dozen red sores the size of half dollars. The clerk said, "Have you considered colonics?"

Susan turned to me and said, "I'm sorry, Scott, but I'll never do colonics."

The thing is, I don't care whether or not somebody does colonics. I said, "Susan, it doesn't matter to me whether you do colonics, but I'm not the one with sores on my legs."

Two months later I received a call from Susan and she is "so desperate that she'll try anything," even colonics. I had no idea whether colonics would help her. I did have clients with skin conditions clear-up after doing colonics, but Susan's case was extreme. I also explained to her all the disclaimers that colonics does not treat disease. And that I've had clients with skin problems not seem to clear.

She did five colonics within ten days. By day #10, every single one of those sores changed from red to pink to pale pink.

Who cares, right? This was just something that Susan and I knew that we knew and that was good enough. No big deal. Some ugly sores gone.

When I was interviewed by *The Tennessean*, the reporter asked to phone some of my clients. I called Susan, since she was a nurse, and asked her permission to be interviewed. She agreed and then I received a call back from her. She said the reporter wanted to quote her and put her *name* in the newspaper.

Put yourself in her shoes -- you are a nurse. The article will say you did colonics and the whole town will also know that you had gross sores on your legs.

I said, "Susan, that's your call."

She replied, "If you think it might help one other person like me, I'll do it."

That's heroism, man. She said yes to them. Her name appeared in the newspaper. The only thing was that the reporter made her improvement from the colonics sound accidental. Like it cleared up "after several months" and she stopped doing colonics. And that's the media.

The point is that Susan sweat bullets over having her name in the newspaper. She gave her PERMISSION to have her name in the newspaper. You don't do that lightly.

Why did she allow that? Because she didn't know she was

constipated before she did colonics. When you are constipated, the small intestine backs up. The liver backs up. The lymphatic system backs up. The skin backs up. When you clean the colon, it helps the skin. Susan just wanted others to know about that simple relationship.

The human body has something else about it besides being flesh and bone. The human body has spaces inside. It has been designed to be hollow. When you cram it full of food all the time, those spaces fill in with gunk. The insides no longer can breathe. Systems begin to clog and fester and rot. All the hollow spaces can fill like an overloaded vacuum cleaner bag.

The net result is disease.

"When you clean the colon, it helps the skin."

How do you know you are constipated? You start showing signs of diseases. You start looking like hell. You get dark puffy circles under the eyes. You feel exhausted in the morning before you even get out of bed. Your skin also starts to flake and rot.

While I am explaining constipation to Gwen, the colonic tubing begins to shudder and we see a gusher of brown poop mixed in orange water rush from her body. End to end, she releases about four feet of solid poop.

The other point I tell Gwen about constipation is that I am a colon hygienist. We see what comes out all day long. If Americans have become generally constipated, a colon hygienist would have a reason for forming an opinion. A fairly qualified opinion.

I try not to, but I can't help myself. "If you're not constipated," I ask her, "Then where did all that poop just come from?"

The impending great divorce

My friend and mentor, Guy Avery, told me that when a business reaches the height of its prosperity, it should begin leaning toward the next wave of opportunity. For example, at the time the first airplane was flown at Kitty Hawk, railroads were at their peak. If the railroad men had been more keen, they could have invested in the Wright brothers.

Now, with the high cost of petro-fuel, airlines might consider investing in railroads. Follow what Nissan Motors advertising says, "Shift, change, adapt."

When fast food was at its peak, the masses were virtually unaware of diet's role in health. Now there is at least one major motion picture, *Super Size Me*, documenting a person's deteriorating health in relation to fast food consumption. And when the U.S. government starts protecting an industry against litigation, that means it's leaking badly. The fast food industry can either fight the truth and a losing battle, or they can change and realign. Profits and truth always go hand-in-hand.

"If the veggies don't vibrate on their own merit, don't bother serving them."

The challenge is that fast food created fast food farming and Franken-farming. That will be an ugly divorce, but divorce it must to survive. Organic is the future. If the veggies don't vibrate on their own merit, don't bother serving them.

The pharmaceutical industry faces the exact same challenges. You can't keep peeing in the pool and inviting folks in because "the water is fine." Slight of hand does reach a point of diminishing returns. Try as you might, we are not the former Soviet Union where every official was on the take.

We do have the media. For a while it appeared that its stealth was for reporting the party line, but that's changed -- somewhat. The Internet is an interesting news source, like www.truthout.com.

Any American citizen reading www.bushwatch.com would have known U.S. troops wouldn't find WMDs long before the Iraq war. Watch independent documentary films like "The Corporation." It's newsworthy stuff. I watch Bill O'Reilly sometimes also to see what's going on in the minds of America.

Inside Poop has introduced concepts that you don't hear much anywhere. The discussion of our national health care problems has been side-tracked as a crisis of insurance, while the discussion needs to refocus on our national HEALTH. Folks with cancer might thank God if they are covered by insurance, but it's way better to thank God that you're not sick at all. That would be the end-in-mind for our nation, wouldn't it?

Anyway, we were talking about money. And that certain corporate ventures can't continue basing profits on the stupidity of the public. Adolf Hitler attempted that very same thing, and I'm sorry, but you will always end up in a bunker with a gun to your own head when you push such foolery to its limits.

Ask the makers of Vioxx about that.

There is a line in the Bible which says, "The hunter sets his net in full view of the birds." American corporations have operated long enough under the mentality of hidden agenda. What's happening today is that the radical ideas of Jesus are just now filtering into the business models of making a profit. It took about two thousand years. Another name for it is integrity. It comes with peace of mind built-in.

The reason that the "quality" movement (T.Q.M.) petered-out can be traced to the fact that those at the bottom of the hierarchy saw through it for what it was -- more manipulative hype. Tell me that the mention of "exceeding expectations" doesn't turn your stomach. Integrity happens while others aren't noticing. And not only that, understand that Jesus sleeps with one eye watching over you. If that has you laughing, I'm laughing right there with you.

Caesar never was cool, and if you are paying attention, that realization is the future.

In the future

Already, corporations are responding to the public awareness that organic is better. How so? Corporations have influenced the government of the United States to change guidelines defining what organic means. Certain corporations like Kraft foods and Wal-Mart, want *in* on the growth of the organic foods industry, which has been growing at ten times the rate of traditional grocery sales -- a 20 percent annual growth compared to two-percent.

Because top level corporate executives have no concept of what organic food even is, they want to label their food as organic too. However, they don't think they need to change how the crops are raised or processed. Instead, they seek to only change the label. In other words, our public officials voted into office are helping to fool the very public they represent. Jesus named these people for what they were -- whitewashed on the outside while on the inside they are full of dead men's bones. If they have their way, the term "organic" will be meaningless, whitewashed, and dead.

"Certain corporations like Kraft foods and Wal-Mart, want *in* on the growth of the organic foods industry."

Check this with the Organic Consumer's Union at www.OrganicConsumers.com.

Another response of growth in a particular sector is to regulate it. Twenty years ago, the massage therapy industry was in its infancy and few states regulated it. Now most states have a board regulating and licensing a massive massage industry.

The State of Tennessee has a massage licensure program and I entered into it as licensee #1100. After I worked at a day spa for two years, I quit. Shortly thereafter, my employer phoned me to come work on a temporary basis filling in for therapists calling in sick. One of the clients I then massaged claimed I pulled the sheet off of her body and massaged her breasts. I did not do this and was dumbfounded by her accusations.

I was interviewed by a State health board investigator and several times during my explanation she said, "You shouldn't have done that!" Stuff like "massage the stomach" or "stretch the legs," which I was trained in massage school to perform. Finally I asked the investigator if she ever had experienced a massage and she said, "No."

Still, I received a letter in the mail saying that I was being charged with sexual misconduct. I phoned the secretary for the massage board to see if my licensure provided me with a legal defense. No, it did not.

I approached a few former employees of the day spa to ask if they might speak on my behalf as to my character. Three-out-of-three said no. When I asked why, I discovered that each had already been sued by the owner of the day spa after they quit and then launched their own business. They were afraid of more retributions. I asked one former staffer if she thought I was being framed and her reply was, "Most likely."

I defended myself against the charges without an attorney and won the case. The girl who made claims was such a bad liar it baffled me that the case even made it to court. The massage board attended to the case for at least six hours that day. I discovered then, what the system of licensure offered me, the therapist, was not one single ounce of benefit and certainly no apologies.

The entire focus of the licensure board is to prosecute their own members. I called it taxation without representation. Never mind a vindictive employer or other vested interests -- onward to the prosecution!

But I got through it and then over it.

Colon hygiene has minimal regulations and should stay that way. Once regulating bodies get involved, the whole thing gets dumber. The ones who would want to control colon hygiene are the same ones who believe it competes with their bottom line. Once they gain regulative control, they will be closer to their goal of squashing it.

The industry of colonics on the whole is not harming people. I believe the record of colonics stands that **not one** case of litigation has proven that any harm occurred from a colonic treatment.

Medicine should consider its own record and realize that it plays within a glass house. The very lowest number of DEATHS from hospital errors is 45,000 annually. The high estimate is 200,000. Call it collateral damage or simply bad homeland security. What would you call it?

"Medicine should consider its own record and realize that it plays within a glass house."

Some critics of my material will point out that Adelle Davis was proven wrong on lots of health advice and that she herself was a victim of cancer. Let the critics disprove the Adelle Davis quotes I have used here. I mean, let the critics disprove me on any of my points. I am always open to change my understanding, always, but will never deny what I have seen with my own eyes.

The future of health in America will require that people are free to cleanse their bodies as they have been doing for THOUSANDS OF YEARS. Pay attention if suddenly the media grabs hold of a single case where a person "was killed or injured" from a colonic. Realize that at this very moment somebody just took a pill in America and keeled over dead from an adverse reaction. And about ten others just now suffered from a drug reaction that impaired their health, function, and happiness.

The basic rule of thumb is that medicine has become controlled by layers of money and alternative health practitioners prefer not getting that political. Everybody I know in colon hygiene prefers to fly low and avoid attention from the controlling social element with their layers of bias and paperwork.

Once politics gets involved, expect lies. Once the media takes the lead, expect sensationalism. Maybe that will change. I hope so.

I envision a future of prospering small farmers once again drawing close to the land. A tomato plant with ripening fruit can't lie nor create sensationalism. The further we get from the cell phone towers, the better. It's a fairly simple truth. I am not sure how it will transition, but hopefully the hired-hand bureaucrats will keep their mitts off while the rest of us slink off into the fields and amongst the trees.

I am not suggesting to abandon the cities behind their bristling levees. What I am saying is that I have a dream. What's yours? I'd hope to see some crazy entrepreneur, like Ray Kroc, start a chain of restaurants that will make only raw, organic meals served on a raw, organic bun. What do you want to see? Join me there in that place.

"To know even one life has breathed easier because you have lived, this is to have succeeded."

In the future, the goal will not be to grow old and outlast the battery of your car, but to fully live. That means terror holds no grip as fascination leads us into the unknown. Listen to the poets. For freedom to march it must have honest reasons to be brave. For you and me and nobody else. Are we that brave?

I have felt like marching and it feels like truth burning in the night.

Follow the words of Ralph Waldo Emerson: "Miracles come to the miraculous, not to the arithmetician. They who affect our imagination, the men (and women) who could not make their hands meet around their objects, the rapt, the lost, the fools of ideas -- they suggest what they cannot execute. They speak to the ages, and are heard from afar. Speak what you think now in hard words and tomorrow speak what tomorrow thinks in hard words again, though it contradict everything you said today."

Emerson is also remembered for admonishing us "to leave the world a bit better, whether by a healthy child, a garden patch, or a redeemed social condition; to know even one life has breathed easier because you have lived, this is to have succeeded."

A million sermons have pronounced that the war has been won. Let us stand in line with that ultimate victory. We can then forget striving and turn the battle over to God.

To those who want to recklessly fight, and kill, and maim, to help bring on Armageddon -- back off! For every weapon you have formed, somebody somewhere has already grown a flower. The harder we would strive to deliver judgment, the faster our anger, our fear, and our harsh medicines just killed us off.

A single act of charity or the trading of forgiveness draws us toward a better tomorrow. So -- the only way to succeed, is to join together. Two roads diverge and there is a choice required. In the future, I believe, good and honest ideas will be heard and welcomed with open arms.

The future is now. It's just not widely distributed yet.

The Adventure

Words by Joseph Campbell
Compiled by Guy Avery

The privilege of a lifetime is being who you are.
What you have to do, do as you would play.

You must be willing to get rid of the life you've planned
if you are to have the life that is waiting for you.

Live from your own center and follow your own bliss.
Social expectations will always be the enemy of the individual adventure.
You will need to quit the 'old place' as a snake sheds yesterday's skin.
Keep in mind, there is no security in following the call to adventure,
but nothing is exciting if you know what the outcome will be.

Enter the forest at the darkest point, where there is no path.
If there already is a path, it is not your path; it is someone else's.
If you follow someone else's path,
you will never realize your own unique potential.

As you proceed through life, following your own path,
birds will shit on you.
Don't bother to brush it off -- Instead laugh it off.
Having a sense of humor will give you the spiritual distance you need.

It is by going down into the abyss that you recover the treasures of your life.
Wherever you stumble, there probably lies your treasure.
The very cave you are afraid to enter,
turns out to be the source of what you are looking for.
The damned thing in the cave that was so dreaded becomes your center.

The purpose of the journey is compassion,
and the goal is to bring your treasure back to the world.

About the author

Scott W. Webb has a bachelor's degree in philosophy from Wheaton College in Chicago. He has been a licensed massage therapist since 1998 and for the past five years has built a thriving private practice as a colon hygienist. He lives with his two teenagers in Nashville, Tennessee.

CPSIA information can be obtained
at www.ICGtesting.com
Printed in the USA
FSOW02n2348220116
16054FS